How to be Gorgeous

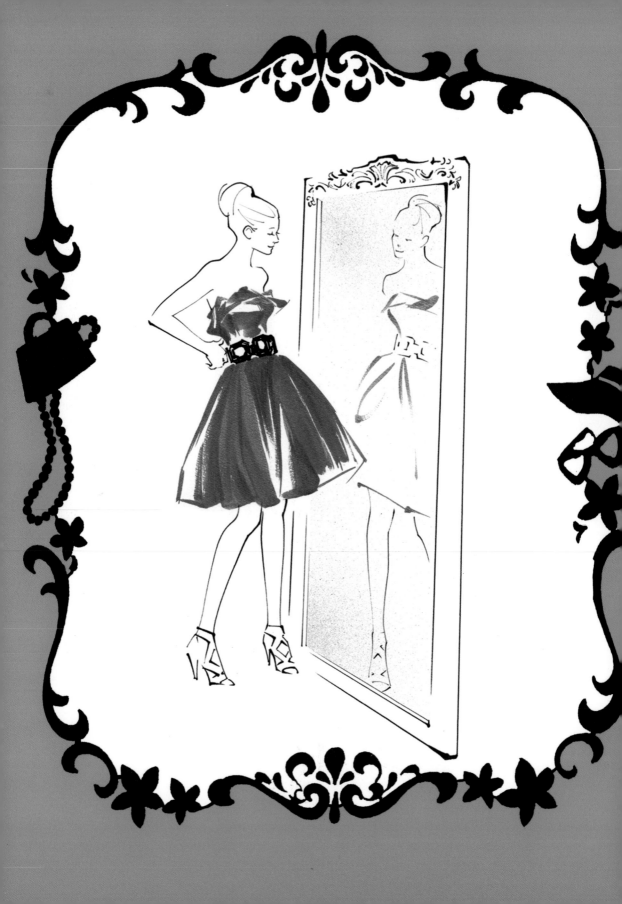

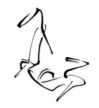

How to be Gorgeous

Wear It Your Way and Feel
Like a *Goddess* Every Day

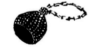

NICKY HAMBLETON-JONES

Photography by Neil Cooper and Illustrations by Yoco

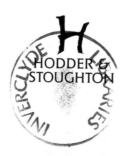

HODDER & STOUGHTON

First published in Great Britain in 2010 by Hodder & Stoughton
An Hachette UK company

1

A CIP catalogue record for this title is available from the British Library

ISBN 978 0340 924150

Photography © Neil Cooper
Illustration © Yoco/ Dutch Uncle

Additional photographic sources:
Benoît Audureau: 17, 32, 50, 57, 73, 93, 114, 133, 155, 157, 194, 217, 218.
Getty Images: Carlos Alvarez 17, Richard E. Aaron 37, Eric Ryan 57, Toru Yamanaka 79, John
Kobal Foundation 99, Jason LaVeris 119, Tim Graham 139, Kevin Winter 181, Jon Furniss 201.

Art Directed and Designed by Nikki Dupin
Typeset in MYRIAD and OONA
Printed and bound by Graficas Estella, Spain

Hodder & Stoughton policy is to use papers that are natural, renewable and recyclable
products and made from wood grown in sustainable forests. The logging and
manufacturing processes are expected to conform to the environmental
regulations of the country of origin.

Hodder & Stoughton Ltd
338 Euston Road
London NW1 3BH
www.hodder.co.uk

To my gorgeous hubby Rob,
whose love and support make
anything possible.

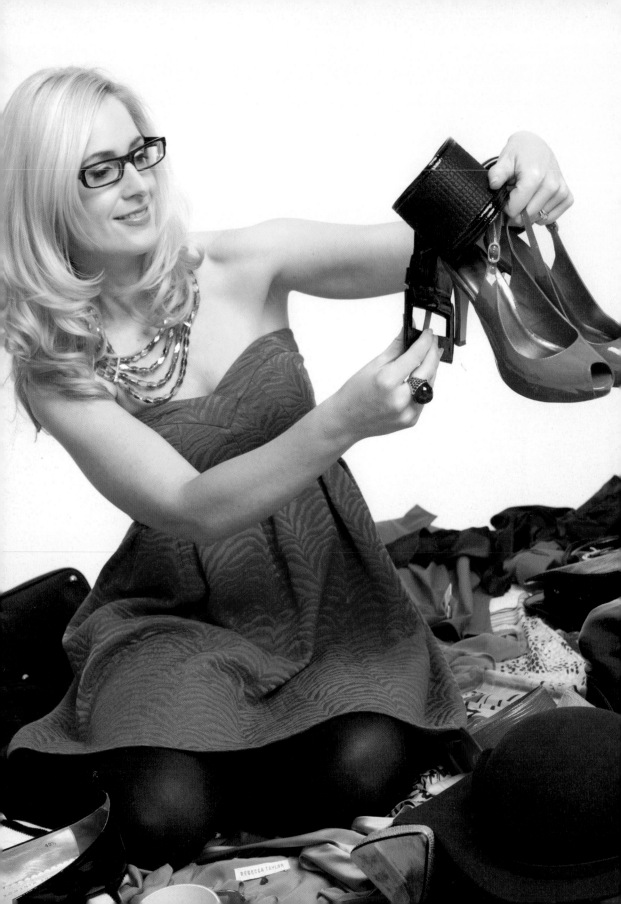

Contents

'STYLE IS SUCH A PERSONAL THING. DON'T WORRY ABOUT WEARING THE LATEST TREND. WORK WITH WHAT YOU'VE GOT. FOCUS ON YOUR BEST BITS.'

Cheryl Cole

YOU ARE A GODDESS. YOU MIGHT NOT KNOW IT YET. YOU MIGHT THINK OF YOURSELF AS A PLAIN JANE, BUT I CAN ASSURE YOU THAT EACH AND EVERY ONE OF US HAS THE POTENTIAL TO LOOK AND FEEL EFFORTLESSLY GORGEOUS.

This is my guide to showing you how. Think of it as having a personal stylist all to yourself. Whether you're after a signature style or a different look for every day of the week, I'll show you where to start, what you need to shop for, where to save money, and how to combine everything with effortless chic.

Keeping up with the changing fashions on the high street can be a time-consuming and sometimes costly endeavour. It can also make you feel bad

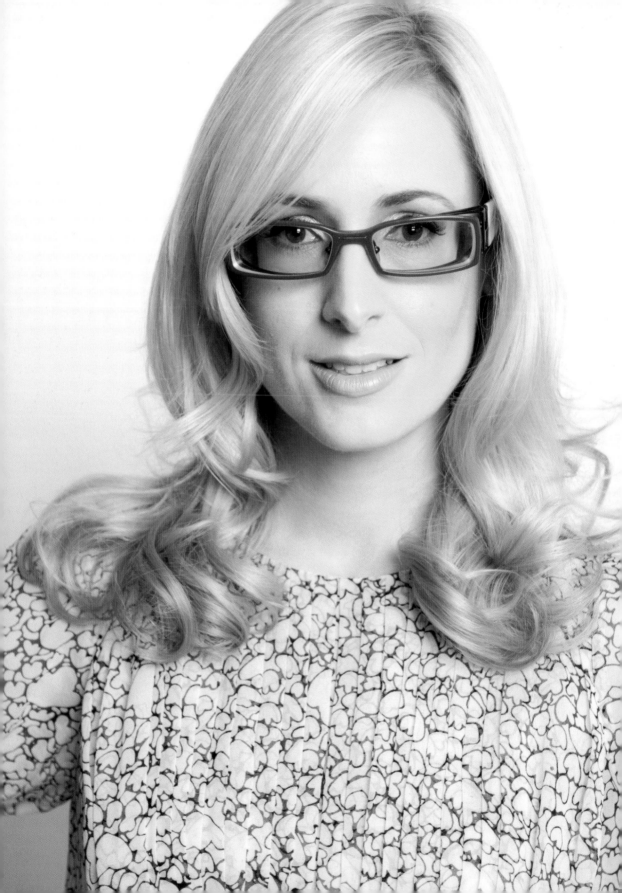

about not ever finding that perfect fit, or clothes that you really love and that represent who you are. How often have you complained that you never have anything to wear, and been tempted to run to the nearest store for that instant fashion fix?

THINK OF SHOPPING LIKE EATING: why fill up on fast food when you could be putting the perfect ingredients together to cook up something really delicious? *How to be Gorgeous* is designed to be a fashion cookbook, showing you how to do just that. Taking a step back from your wardrobe, and using this book to identify what look you really want to create will enable you to develop a more focused, fulfilling approach to how you dress. No more last-minute panic attacks or expensive mistakes! Instead you'll have a range of flattering outfits, not to mention beautiful accessories that'll inject versatility into your wardrobe and give you that head-to-toe wow factor.

It all starts with **TEN ICONIC TRENDS** that will change your life. I've been styling women of all shapes and sizes for many years, and in my experience most of us have a pretty good sense of our body shape and how to conceal our bad bits. But understanding which styles suit us, and pulling a complete look together, top to toe? That still feels like a challenge.

Many women who come to see me tell me they've resorted to wearing a 'uniform' day in, day out – usually jeans and a fleece or T-shirt, accessorised with a flat pair of shoes. Style has been replaced with function. And that's OK (just about!) when you don't have a moment to yourself. But finding a look that expresses your personality and individuality can be truly life-changing and a great makeover is one of the easiest ways to remind yourself (and everyone else) just how sexy, unique and drop-dead fabulous you truly are.

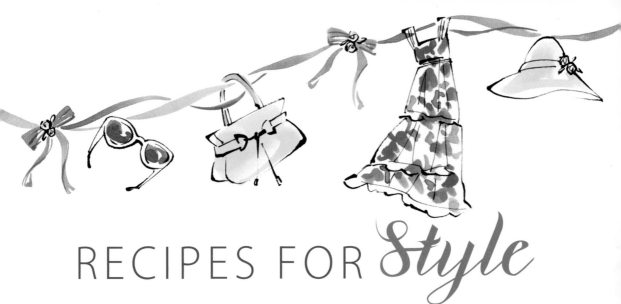

RECIPES FOR *Style*

HOW TO BE GORGEOUS WILL GIVE YOU THE TOOLS AND TECHNIQUES TO EXPRESS YOURSELF, TO HAVE FUN WITH FASHION, AND TO CELEBRATE THE THINGS IN YOURSELF THAT YOU LIKE THE MOST. And just like a cookbook, it will help you put together all sorts of delicious concoctions from a range of fresh, tasty looks.

There is an element of predictability in fashion, which means it is possible to build a wardrobe of items that can be translated into stylish looks year in, year out. That's because modern fashion is more about reinvention than creation. When was the last time something truly revolutionary appeared on the catwalk? Season after season we see the same ideas repackaged. Autumn/winter always has an element of tailoring, tweed, embellishment and luxury. By contrast, spring/summer usually includes a safari or African theme, nautical and floral prints and lots of white punctuated with acid brights.

I want to show you the TOP TEN TRENDS that have stood the test of time and are guaranteed not to date or die an unfashionable death. From TOP GUN to TAILORING, from SPORTS LUXE to VICTORIANA, there's a flattering style to suit every woman and every occasion.

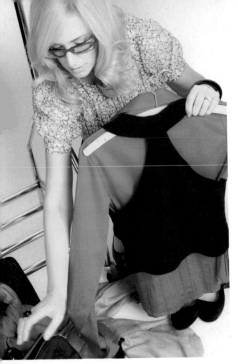

I've broken each look down into its most basic parts, with recipes for style to show you exactly how designers and personal stylists put the look together for maximum effect.

If there are items you need to buy, my lists of ingredients (ten basic items for each look) will make shopping for clothes, or even rifling through your wardrobe, a whole lot easier as you'll know exactly what you're looking for. You won't need to buy a lot. Many basics can be adapted to suit a number of looks. And sometimes it's just a case of adapting what you have, and buying a few key accessories.

I've listed the trimmings that will give you that all-important fashionable edge and included tips on how to adapt each look for your body shape, for different occasions, and from season to season. There's also a masterclass on hair and make-up at the end of each chapter, packed with professional styling secrets, and a 'get gorgeous' shopping guide at the end of the book to help you source the best styling products and most covetable cosmetic goodies.

I have included some dos and don'ts to give you guidance. But as your confidence grows, please feel free to experiment. If you don't like them, break, bend or ignore any rules I mention along the way, and discover what works for you. I want this book to stimulate not suffocate your sense of style and self-expression, so remember that no one became a Style Icon by following the rules. Once you've mastered the basics, you should work out how to wear it your way. You'll be amazed at how many options you have!

WHAT'S YOUR *Look?*

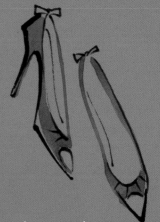

Use *How to be Gorgeous* to find one look that really stands out and translates well across all aspects of your lifestyle, or to help you create a repertoire of looks so that you can adopt a different style every day of the week. For example, a TAILORED look might be ideal for the office, with a BOHO twist for the weekend and a touch of DISCO for a girls' night out.

HERE ARE SOME SIMPLE TIPS TO SET YOU ON YOUR WAY:

✦ Go through the book and pick out a few looks that appeal to you.

✦ Check through the key ingredients for each look.

✦ Go through your existing wardrobe and cross off any of the ingredients you already own.

✦ Do the same with your accessories.

✦ Then go through the styling suggestions chart for each look and pick out three combinations that appeal to you. Use these to further narrow down your wish list.

✦ This is about building up a wardrobe for life. Don't try and buy everything now! Keep a list of the items you're looking out for and update each season.

NOW LET THE TRANSFORMATION BEGIN!

chapter 1

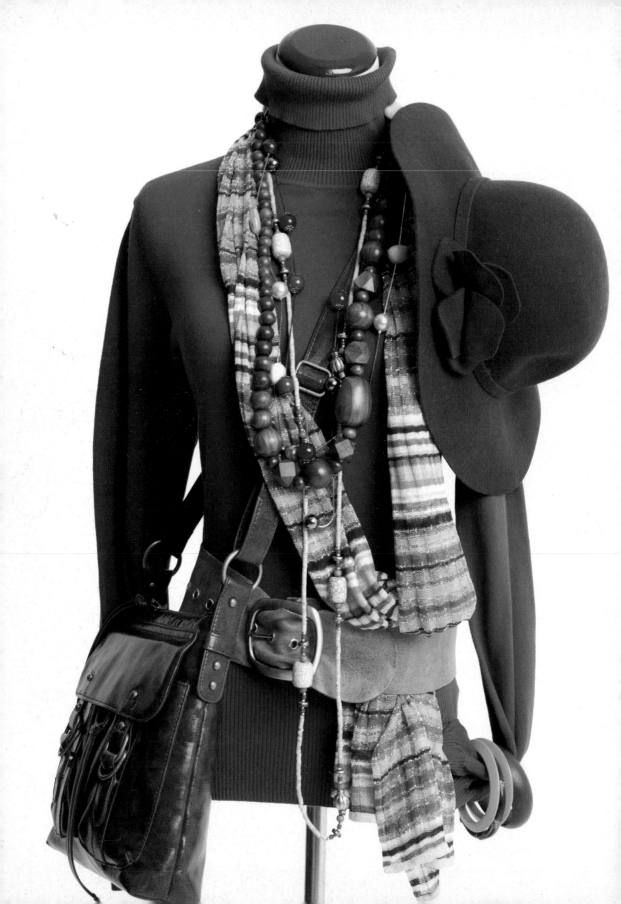

Boho

YOU CAN BE A FREE SPIRIT AND LOOK MODERN AND SEXY. A LOT MORE THAN KAFTANS, COIN-BELTS AND GYSPY SKIRTS, BOHO IS A PRACTICAL, FEMININE LOOK THAT CAN BE ADOPTED BY EASY-GOING *Goddesses* OF ANY AGE.

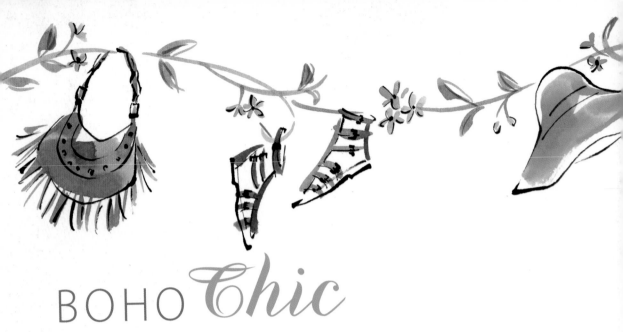

BOHO *Chic*

OWING MUCH TO THE HIPPIE STYLES OF THE 1960S, BOHO HAS BEEN A HUGE TREND THROUGHOUT THE NOUGHTIES. This look is a perfect balance of intended messiness, artistic creativity and vintage chic. Its use of bright colours and ethnic influences makes for relaxed, easy, fun fashion, and the eclectic layering of simple shapes give an effortlessly feminine style that many women aspire to.

Inspiration FROM THE A-LIST

SIENNA MILLER IS THE INDISPUTABLE 'PRINCESS OF BOHO'. Her signature look, made up of floaty tunics, ethnic jewellery, long peasant skirts, jeans tucked into boots and studded belts, is fresh and stylish. She started the Boho craze by simply throwing together outfits and pairing them with

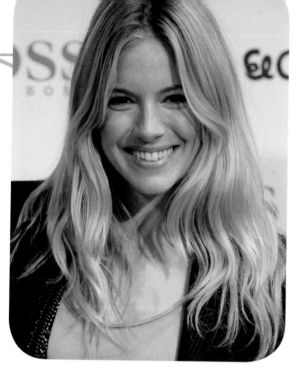

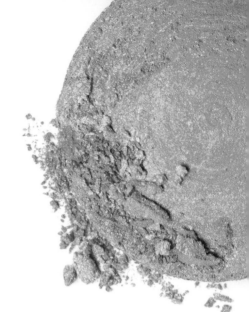

comfortable old favourites, like her Ugg boots. Her wardrobe is filled with a mixture of vintage 60s and 70s pieces fused with modern designer creations and all-important 'It' bags. The whole look is completed with simple make-up, bare lips and flushed cheeks.

Sienna's real art is her ability to layer the most unlikely combinations and restyle a garment in a completely different way. She famously went out one night wearing a black shirt that she borrowed from a friend and wore around her chest with a cropped cardigan. The following day everyone was rushing out to recreate the same look.

'I'M REALLY NOT GOOD AT DRESSING UP AND BEING GLAMOROUS. I'M FINE WHEN I'M JUST WAKING UP AND PUTTING ON A PAIR OF JEANS.'
Sienna Miller

Key INGREDIENTS

WHAT I LOVE ABOUT THIS LOOK IS THAT YOU CAN MAKE UP THE RULES AS YOU GO ALONG. The idea is to create something that's soft and feminine, but still looks fashionable as opposed to frumpy.

1 WEATHERED JEANS

Don't divert too much from the style of **JEANS** that suit you best. Whether you prefer straight, bootleg or skinny jeans, stick with what you like and just opt for something with more of a distressed or 'worn' finish. If you have an old pair of jeans you hardly wear, why not distress them yourself and give them a new lease of life? Simply:

✦ Place a block of wood or an old book inside the trouser leg you want to distress.

✦ Rub a steak knife or cheese grater against the denim. Rub gently for mild distress; rub longer and more vigorously for holes and tears.

✦ Do not cut holes with scissors. This creates a suspiciously un-frayed and consequentially un-stylish effect.

✦ Fray jeans by rubbing sandpaper around pockets, knees, hemlines, or any other area that you want to have a soft, worn appearance.

✦ Dampen a sponge with bleach and rub it around the outer edges of holes for a faded look.

 Tip *Teaming prints with DENIM immediately tones them down and gives them a more youthful edge.*

2 WIDE-LEG TROUSERS

If you're not a huge fan of jeans, slouchy **WIDE-LEG TROUSERS** in neutral shades such as beige, stone or light brown are a great alternative. Make sure you don't overdo volume. Teaming wide-leg trousers with a fitted blouse and a belt, or a blazer layered over a blouse, will keep it soft, feminine and in proportion.

3 PRINTED DRESS

A key element of modern Boho is the **PRINTED DRESS**. This is a great look, particularly if you are self-conscious about your legs. Wearing a dress over jeans or trousers will make it more versatile and give you the confidence to experiment. Alternatively, team with thick tights and flat knee-high boots.

4 BLOUSON TOP

By **BLOUSON** I'm not suggesting something your grandmother would wear, but a sheer/chiffon top with delicate print and bell sleeves. The beauty of a blouson-style top is the voluminous sleeves, making it ideal if you're self-conscious about your bingo wings.

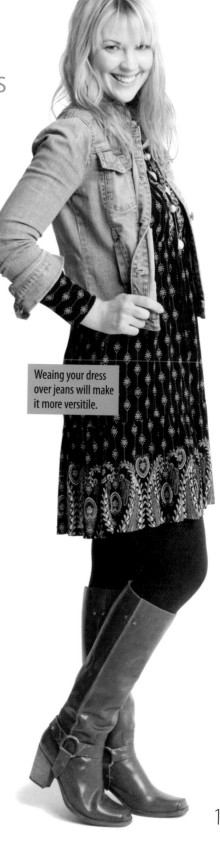

Weaing your dress over jeans will make it more versitile.

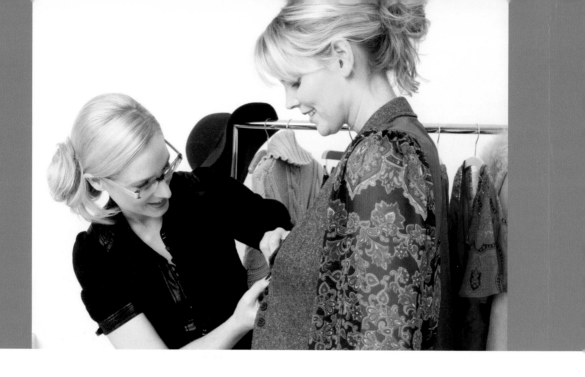

5 TUNICS/KAFTANS WITH EMBROIDERY

Embellishment is another key element of the Boho look. Loose **TUNIC-STYLE TOPS** or **KAFTANS** with detail around the sleeves or neckline are ideal; they hide a multitude of sins and create a striking feature.

> *Tip* *Make sure you create shape and structure by adding a belt or layering under a jacket and remember to balance out proportions.*

6 WAISTCOAT

A **WAISTCOAT** really is an essential piece of your Boho toolkit, simply because it helps to create shape by defining the waist. It is also ageless – anyone can wear a waistcoat, and layering it over printed tops the Boho way makes it infinitely more feminine. Make sure your waistcoat doesn't compete with the print on your top. Opt for something in a neutral colour with minimal embellishment so it creates shape not a statement.

7 LONG-SLEEVED JERSEY TOPS

FINE KNITS or even **T-SHIRTS** are fantastic for layering under dresses and tops or simply over each other to create a more eclectic look. Using layering in this way will also make your wardrobe more wearable throughout the year.

8 DENIM JACKET

A **DENIM JACKET** will always be a great wardrobe staple. Make sure you choose one that nips you in at the waist and isn't too boxy. A softer, worn jacket will give you more of a hip factor – try searching second-hand and vintage shops or perhaps resurrect the old one in your attic.

> *Tip* *Avoid wearing DENIM with denim. If you love your jeans I'd stick to waistcoats and leather or cotton jackets to soften the look.*

9 SOFT STRUCTURED BLAZER

I've included a **BLAZER** because it's another fantastic wardrobe staple that will come in handy whether or not you're having a Boho moment. Fantastic worn over blouson tops and jeans, or teamed with wide-leg trousers for a grown-up, tailored look.

10 TAN VINTAGE-LOOKING BOOTS

By **BOOTS** I'm referring to knee-highs, either flat or with a small heel, that you can either wear under or over your trousers or jeans. These are a stylish alternative for yummy mummies who would otherwise live in their trainers. The older the better – shiny new boots simply won't do. Take them for a walk in the country to put them through their paces.

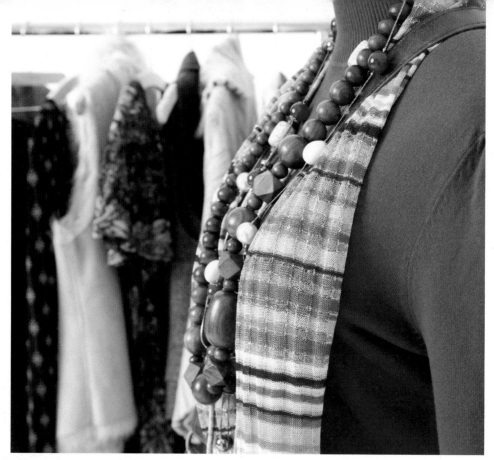

Trimmings

AS WITH ANY LOOK IT'S THE ACCESSORIES THAT REALLY GIVE IT A POINT OF DIFFERENCE AND A STYLISH FLAIR, and when it comes to Boho, the more the merrier! These essential accessories will complement your Boho capsule wardrobe.

✦ LARGE TAN LEATHER BELT
Choose a waisted or hipster BELT depending on your body shape or opt for one of each if you're slim. The wider the better, and interesting buckle detailing is a must.

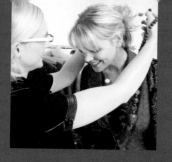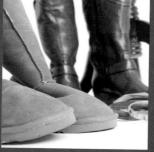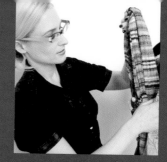

✦ SLOUCHY LEATHER MESSENGER BAG

Not only is this a Boho essential, it's also a practical solution. The long leather strap enables you to wear the BAG slung across the body for a casual but chic look.

✦ ETHNIC SCARF

The thickness of the SCARF depends on your body shape. If you're small-chested, a large cable-knit scarf will set you off for Boho heaven. For something less heavy, opt for an Indian style scarf with tassel detailing worn over your jacket and wrapped around your neck.

✦ CHUNKY BANGLES

Large, chunky wooden BANGLES worn together are ideal if you want to draw attention away from your bingo wings and towards your wrists.

✦ LONG BEADS/NECKLACES

An ideal way to divert attention away from broad shoulders and wide chests and to elongate the body. It's best if you don't compete with print, pattern or embellishment on tops. Wear with plain tops and blouses. With bold prints, opt for earrings or bangles instead.

✦ FLOPPY HAT

Perfect for keeping the sun off your face on a warm spring day while still complementing your overall look.

✦ DANGLY EARRINGS

Long, chandelier-style EARRINGS are perfect for this look, especially if you have long hair. Bejewelled designs in metallics like bronzes and golds are ideal.

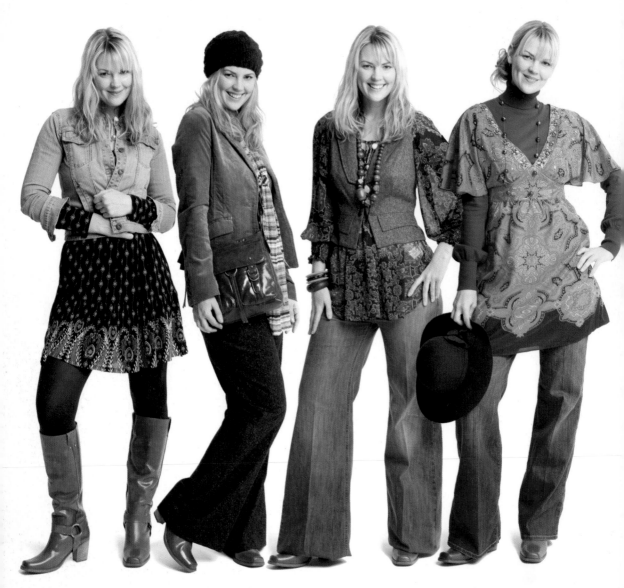

✦ The denim jacket
+ printed dress +
tan heeled boots

✦ The soft structed
blazer + wide leg
trousers

✦ The wide-leg
jeans + waistcoat
+ printed tunic

✦ The printed
tunic + worn jeans
+ floppy hat

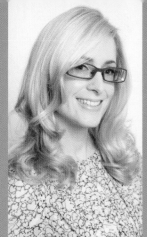

Styling
SUGGESTIONS

	Worn Jeans	Printed Tunic	Waistcoat	Blouson Top	Structured Blazer	Wide-Leg Trousers	Printed Dress	Long-Sleeved Jersey Top	Denim Jacket	*Now...* ACCESSORISE YOUR OUTFIT
1	✓	✓	✓							TAN HEELED BOOTS, CHUNKY BANGLES, MESSENGER BAG
2			✓	✓		✓				TAN HEELED BOOTS, DANGLY EARRINGS, LONG NECKLACE
3						✓	✓	✓		TAN FLAT BOOTS, MESSENGER BAG
4		✓				✓			✓	TAN FLAT OR HEELED BOOTS, TAN BELT, LONG BEADS
5	✓			✓	✓					TAN HEELED BOOTS, TAN BELT, ETHNIC SCARF
6		✓			✓	✓				TAN HEELED BOOTS, LONG BEADS, MESSENGER BAG
7	✓	✓						✓		TAN FLAT BOOTS, TAN BELT, CHUNKY BANGLES
8							✓		✓	TAN FLAT OR HEELED BOOTS, DANGLY EARRINGS
9	✓			✓	✓			✓		TAN HEELED BOOTS, CHUNKY BANGLES, TAN BELT
10			✓			✓		✓		TAN HEELED BOOTS, ETHNIC SCARF, DANGLY EARRINGS

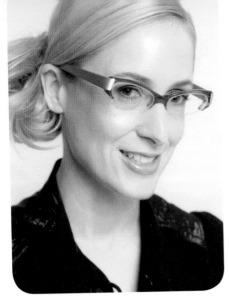

Wear it
YOUR WAY

BOHO SUITS ALL SHAPES AND SIZES, as the principle of layering means that you can highlight your best assets and disguise all the bits you don't like. Here's how to make it work for you:

Pear Shapes
(carry weight on their hips and bum):

✦ Hip-length tunics could not be more suited to a pear shape as they flare out over the hips, covering the bottom but at the same time highlighting the slimness around the upper body.

✦ Look for tops that have detail around the neckline in the form of beading and/or embroidery to take attention away from the hips.

✦ For practicality and warmth, layer a polo neck or a long-sleeved jersey top in a complementary colour under a soft fabric tunic top or dress and belt at the waist. Team with a pair of dark denim bootleg jeans.

Apple Shapes
(carry weight on their tummy and chest):

✦ Go for a long slouchy cardigan over a simple blouse and wear a low-slung belt around cardigan. Arrange so that a slice of top underneath

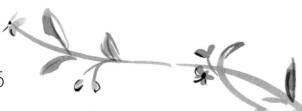

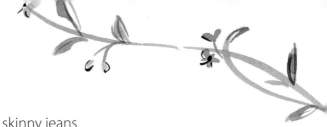

can be seen and team with skinny jeans.

- Wear a long kaftan-style top with bold prints. This will disguise lumps and bumps and elongate the body at the same time.

Hourglass
(curvaceous all over with a small waist):

- Wear a dress belted at the waist with opaque tights and boots.
- Layer a fitted cardigan over a tunic top with jeans tucked into boots.
- Stick with lower-cut necklines to show off décolletage. Try smocks with square, scoop or V-necks and big voluminous sleeves.

Boy/Straight *(tall and lacking in curves):*

- Wear skinny jeans tucked into boots and go for fitted, softly tailored blazers with camisole-style tops and accessorise with long gold chains.
- Pair a smock dress with a cute belt to create curves, or dress it down with an open, fitted waistcoat and skinny jeans.
- Get a simple vest and team with a floor-sweeping gypsy skirt and a low-slung heavy leather belt.

Strawberry Shaped
(broad shoulders and a wide back):

- Go for low-neckline tops and wear with big chunky bangles to draw focus down the arm. Wear with jeans tucked into boots.
- Look for tunics that have detail towards the bottom half to draw the eye down the body. Avoid too much ruffle detailing around neckline.
- Go for tops with flared bell-shape sleeves to soften shoulders.

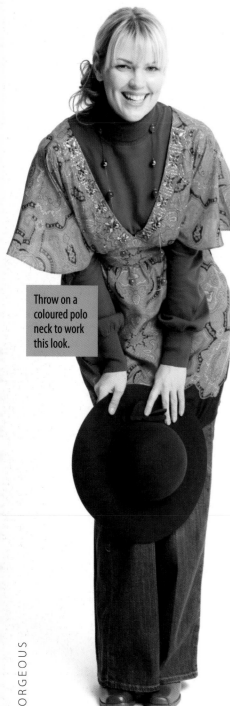

Throw on a coloured polo neck to work this look.

Seasoning

BEING ABLE TO ADAPT YOUR LOOK THROUGH THE SEASONS IS GREAT, and will save you money as you won't have to invest in two completely different sets of clothes. Here are some seasonal extras to enable you to look Boho chic all year round:

Spring/Summer

1 FLAT BEADED SANDALS
2 ESPADRILLES
3 SOFT SUEDE-FRINGED BAGS
4 WHITE JEANS
5 LARGE ROUND SUNGLASSES WITH SLIM FRAMES
6 FLOPPY STRAW HAT
7 MAXI-LENGTH SKIRTS/DRESSES
8 SHORT PUFFED-SLEEVED TOPS/T-SHIRTS

Autumn/Winter

1 DARK BLUE JEANS
2 LONG CABLE-KNIT SCARF
3 SOFT BERET-STYLE HAT
4 COLOURED POLO NECKS
5 BLACK/CHOCOLATE LEATHER BELT
6 OPAQUE TIGHTS
7 CHUNKY KNIT CARDIGAN
8 UGG-STYLE BOOTS

RECIPE FOR *Success*

BOHO DOESN'T TRANSLATE INTO A SEXY EVENING LOOK AND IS USUALLY A BIT TOO MESSY FOR THE OFFICE, BUT IT IS GREAT CASUAL DAYWEAR. Just keep it relaxed, cool and quirky and you won't go far wrong. It's the perfect style for:

1. *Lunch with Friends*

Jeans and a pretty smock teamed with a fitted cardigan in a complementary colour will strike the perfect balance.

2. *Low-Key Dinner or Drinks*

Feel relaxed and hip in an empire-line dress over tan boots, or a colourful blouson top worn with a waistcoat and simple flat-fronted trousers. With the dress, leave off the belt unless you wear it across the empire line itself. It's important not to create more than one line across the body.

3. *The School Run*

For mums who want to look stylish at the school gates, keep it simple and wear jeans tucked into flat boots with a simple smock top or tunic. Boho is about mixing colours, patterns and textures together. Black will sap the life out of this, so use neutrals, browns, blues and greens as your base.

4. *Summer Holidays*

Boho is all about mixing and matching, so select items you can team and layer them in alternative ways. Kaftans, smock dresses, belts and floppy hats all make for an easy capsule suitcase. Remember to keep it soft and feminine. Fabrics should be unstructured and only loosely tailored.

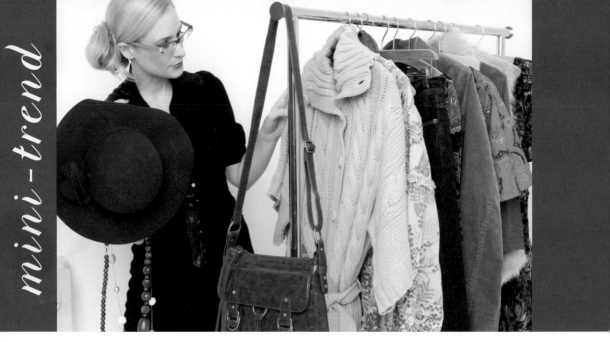

Festival CHIC

CAMPING OUT IN A FIELD means that you can't rely on hair-straighteners or regular showers, but you can count on a fantastic atmosphere where anything goes. Forget the mud . . . here's how to rock a festival, Boho-style.

1 DON'T FORGET YOUR WELLIES – They can be patterned and girly or classic Hunter green, but either way pair them with sexy denim shorts or a short, floaty skirt.

2 HIDE YOUR HAIR – After a couple of shower-free days your tresses aren't going to be at their best, so take the chance to experiment with bandanas, headscarves and hats. A cowboy hat will keep the sun off your face and help your friends spot you in the crowd.

3 ROUGHING IT DOESN'T MEAN LOOKING ROUGH – Even at Glastonbury Kate Moss sparks style trends. Follow her lead and combine a flirty sundress with oversized sunglasses for unbeatable festival chic.

FINISHING TOUCHES

Make-Up Masterclass

BOHO EPITOMISES NATURAL HIPPY CHIC. In make-up terms that translates into a fresh, pretty glow which looks as if you haven't tried too hard – easier said than done! The key to the natural look is to ensure your skin is well moisturised and hydrated before you start.

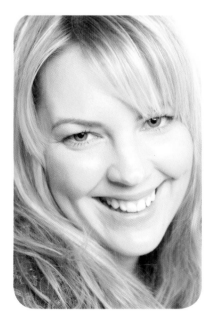

1. Dewy Foundation

To truly emulate Boho beauty, skin needs to look fresh, youthful and dewy. This is easily achieved at any age by using a luminous skin primer and foundation.

- ✦ Mix the illuminating primer with your foundation and apply in thin, even layers over your face.
- ✦ For women over 30, avoid putting foundation on the outer eye, as the foundation will emphasise fine laughter lines.

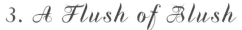

2. Natural Eyes

Pretty, fresh and subtle – Boho babes take make-up inspiration from Mother Nature.

✦ Begin by using your fingers to blend a light-reflecting concealer in the inner corner of your eye.

✦ Using a neutral colour such as a soft pink or brown, apply by sweeping it across the eyelid and blend.

3. A Flush of Blush

Once you've created a gorgeous dewy foundation, it is essential that you use a cream blush. This will slide easily over your dewy foundation and has a lovely youthful sheen; brilliant if you suffer from dull, lacklustre skin.

✦ Delicately apply the cream blush using your fingers; starting on the apples of your cheeks, blend upward and outwards.

✦ Build up colour gradually by applying in thin layers.

✦ Don't overindulge in product or you risk looking like a clown!

3. Soft Succulent Lips

Use a lipstick stain rather than lashings of lipstick. The trick here is to look as though you aren't really wearing any!

✦ Select a sheer colour that's just one or two shades darker than your natural lip colour .

✦ Create a lipstick stain by dabbing the lipstick onto your lips, then smudge your lips together and blot away the excess.

Drop Dead Hair

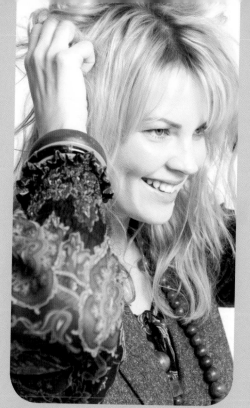

FOR THE QUINTESSENTIAL BOHO LOOK, hair needs to reflect the clothes – relaxed and not over-styled!

1. Short to Medium-Length Hair

✦ Add subtle highlights around your face. Choose one or two shades lighter than your natural hair colour, in order to achieve a natural look.

✦ Soften your fringe by blow-drying your hair using your fingers to mould, style, tousle and give lift to the roots.

✦ Complete the look with a light texturising pomade or serum to define layers and create a soft choppy look.

2. Long Hair

✦ Part your hair in the middle and apply a strong-hold mousse.

✦ Tip your head upside down and use a diffuser to dry your hair.

✦ When dry, tip your hair back and spritz with a non-frizz spray.

✦ Wear loose or softly tied into a low ponytail.

chapter 2

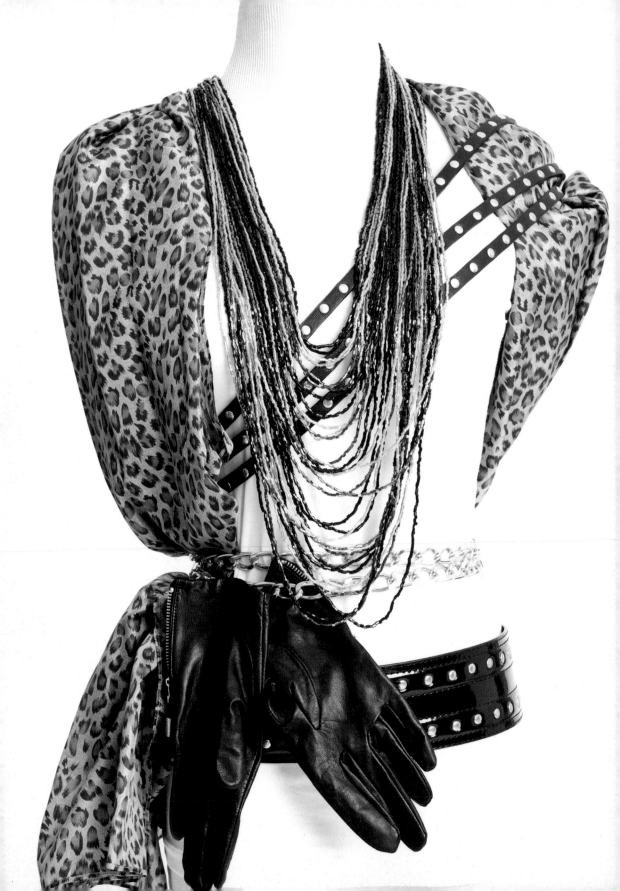

ROCK
Chick

IF YOU'RE WILD AT HEART, ROCK OUT WITH
THIS SUPER-SEXY STYLE THAT'LL HAVE THEM
SCREAMING FOR MORE!

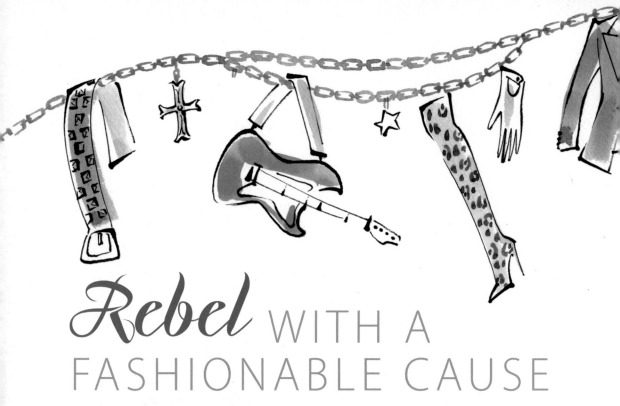

Rebel WITH A FASHIONABLE CAUSE

AN ICONIC STYLE FOR REBELS OF ALL AGES, THIS LOOK IS COOL, SEXY, IRREVERENT, AND HAS BEEN A FASHION STAPLE SINCE THE DAYS OF THE ROLLING STONES. Of course it's not just for rockers. Sid Vicious may have been the first to wear safety pins in his clothes, but Versace made the look ultra-chic. Just think of Liz Hurley at the premiere of *Four Weddings and a Funeral* in that little black dress!

Styled in the right way, this look can breathe new life into a functional wardrobe. The trick is to keep it simple; don't try to emulate the Sex Pistols or Madonna – just be yourself. Adding the odd quirky item like a pair of fishnets or a slim, studded belt is a great place to start. Since there is not a huge amount of colour or print in the **ROCK CHICK**'s wardrobe, the smallest of accessories can be key to creating the overall look. Garments are predominantly fitted and at times revealing, so go for subtlety with just a hint of rock goddess shining through.

Inspiration
FROM THE A-LIST

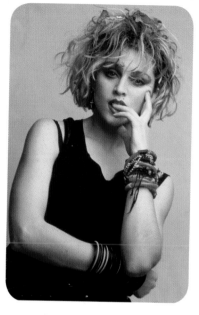

IN THE 1980S, DEBBIE HARRY WAS THE ORIGINAL ROCK CHICK. Like a subversive Marilyn Monroe, she made it OK to be beautiful and bad at the same time. There was always a thrown-together feel to her outfits. Skinny jeans and slinky jersey dresses were teamed with dark sunglasses, white-hot peroxide bob and heavy, studded accessories to create her signature hard-edged glam look. A resourceful approach to style inspired her to add her own twist – a beret or thigh-high boots – to make any outfit into a very sexy statement.

And then there was **MADONNA** writhing on stage in ripped T-shirts and chains. Madonna popularised the gothic look with her love of lace and endless necklaces, crosses, ribbons piled on top of each other. She never looked as if she was trying too hard, and that's how fashion icons are born.

'I THINK YOU CAN BE DEFIANT AND REBELLIOUS AND STILL BE STRONG AND POSITIVE.'
Madonna

Key INGREDIENTS

EVEN FASHION REBELS NEED TO MAKE INVESTMENTS. This look relies particularly heavily on good staple items that you can wear all year round.

1 BLACK/GREY (SKINNY) JEANS

A wardrobe staple. Think Kate Moss in her grey **SKINNY JEANS** teamed with white T-shirt and black pinstripe waistcoat. If you're curvy, opt for straight or bootleg jeans – as long as they're relatively fitted on the thighs you'll still be able to give them a Rock Chick edge. Skinny jeans are also fantastic for layering under jumpers or dresses as they cling to the leg and therefore don't look bulky layered underneath.

2 CROPPED BLACK LEATHER JACKET

A **BIKER JACKET** is a fantastic wardrobe staple and worth investing in. Traditionally these have mandarin collars, and lots of zips, but a stylish cropped leather jacket, that's belted or fitted in the waist, will also do the trick. Whatever style you choose, make sure it's shaped in the waist and not too boxy.

3 FITTED WHITE SHIRT

From sexy dress shirts to pretty smocked styles, this classic piece comes in many delightful guises and will forever be a style staple. If you already own a few basic white shirts, why not opt for something different: exaggerated collars or cuffs, ruffle detailing or pussy bows are all great alternatives.

4 FAVOURITE ROCK BAND T-SHIRT

A mainstay of Rock Chick regalia, **ROCK BAND T-SHIRTS** can look fab, but make sure yours is fitted. If it's vintage, a little fading can add to the coolness, but make sure it's not grubby!

> *Tip* *If you don't own one already, go for something with a strong motif or logo on it. The bolder the better: it needs to make a statement about you.*

5 HIGH-WAISTED SLIM-LEG TROUSERS

If you lived through the 80s, you're probably horrified at the thought of having to wear Olivia Newton-John suck-on trousers again. As painful as they may have been first time round, you'll probably find them a lot more comfortable now. Love-em or hate-em, **HIGH-WAISTED TROUSERS** do wonders for your legs. Black is the most practical colour to invest in. Always team with high heels to make your legs look longer.

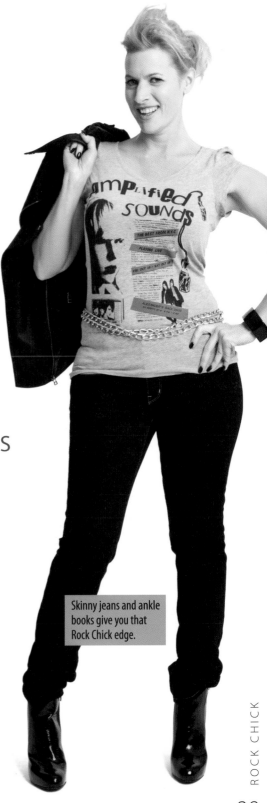

Skinny jeans and ankle boots give you that Rock Chick edge.

6 SLINKY BLACK DRESS

This needs to be strong and sexy, so look for one that is fitted and knee-length – mid-thigh will look 'rock cheap', rather than chic. Choose between a flattering slash neck or a low neckline for real sex appeal, and accessorise with a black patent belt round the waist.

7 FITTED BLACK WAISTCOAT

Ever see a rocker without a **WAISTCOAT?** Single breasted waistcoats are more versatile and easy to wear. Wear closed, over loose shirts and baggy Ts to create shape, or open over fitted shirts and vest tops for a more casual look.

8 STRAPPY/HALTERNECK TOPS IN BOLD COLOURS

I think it's a given that animal print should not be worn by anyone over the age of 40 – unless you've got the pizzazz to carry it off. Polka dots and stripes, on the other hand, are easy to wear at any age and add a fun feminine aspect to what is in essence quite a masculine look.

> *Tip* *HALTERNECK and STRAPPY TOPS are often difficult to wear as we get older. Layering under a jacket will make them versatile.*

9 PLUNGING V-NECK SWEATER

This can be worn day or night and dressed up or down. Regardless of body shape, make sure yours is fitted and hip length. A black **SWEATER** is essential but a couple in bright block colours such as red or blue will help break up the monochrome.

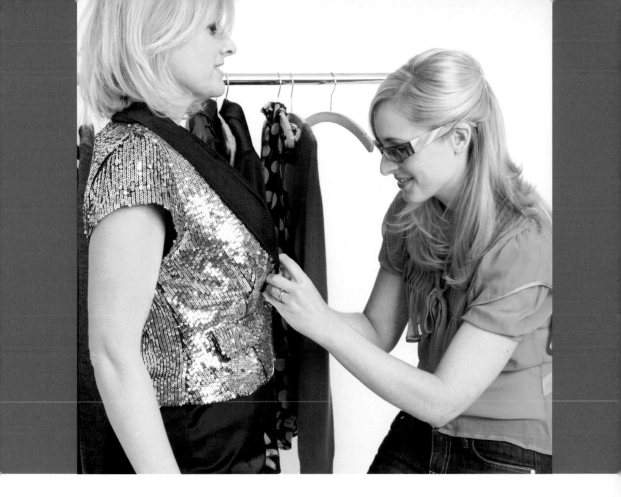

10 TUXEDO JACKET

Perfect for when you want to look cool but low-key. If you've forgotten to shave your legs, simply team a **TUX JACKET** with high-waisted trousers or jeans and a fitted white shirt and you're sure to hit the right note.

> *Tip* *If you prefer to invest in a suit, choose the TUXEDO by the shape of the trousers. Whether you favour flares, straight high-waisters or super-skinny cigarette pants, this is a look that will work any time, any place, anywhere.*

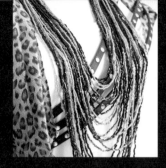
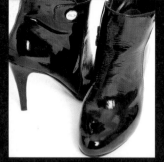
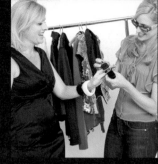

Trimmings

ACCESSORIES ARE A KEY PART OF THIS LOOK. Listed below are some key pieces to inspire you to get your rocks on!

✦ STUDDED BELT

Metallic detailing on belts, bags and bracelets immediately toughens up a look.

✦ LEATHER CUFF/CUT-OUT GLOVES

Although Madonna still manages to carry them off when she's performing, for most of us I think classic black leather gloves or a statement black plastic bracelet CUFF is the closest we should get to cut-outs.

✦ HEAVY CHAINS

Perfect if you're 21, but not so cool if you're 41! A more modern twist would be to wear a chunky necklace with interesting metallic beaded detail.

✦ PATENT LEATHER POINTED ANKLE BOOTS

This is a fantastic way to inject some sex appeal into this look. Patent leather adds shine and interest without too much competing detail. The pointed toe is essential as it will help lengthen the leg. To keep patent leather at its best, spray a little bit of furniture polish onto a cloth and buff lightly.

✦ CHUNKY MONOCHROME BRACELETS

An easy, cost-effective way to modernise your look.

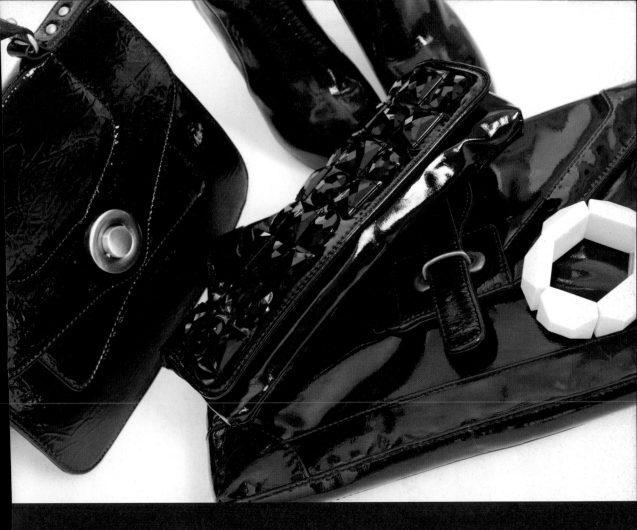

◆ PATENT LEATHER CLUTCH BAG

Whether you've decided to embrace this look or not, a BLACK PATENT
CLUTCH BAG will always be an excellent investment.

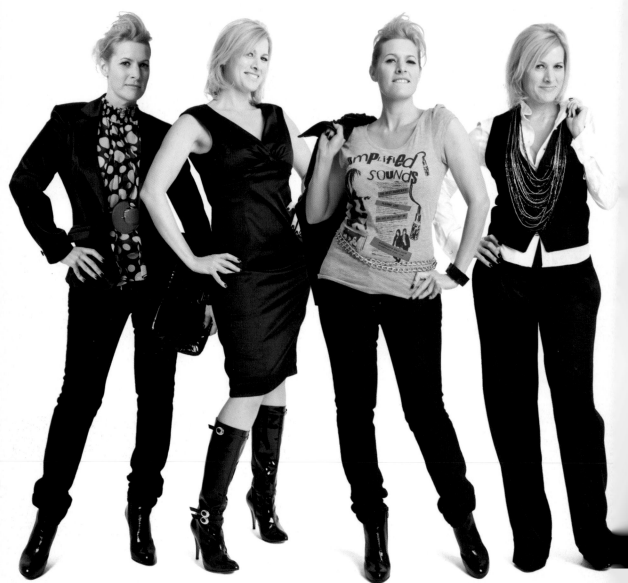

✦ The tuxedo jacket + skinny jeans + patent clutch

✦ Slinky black dress + high heeled patent pointy boots

✦ The rocker T-shirt + skinny jeans + biker jacket

✦ The high-waisted trousers + waistcoat + long necklaces

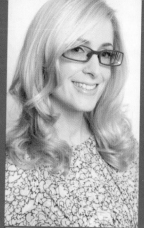

Styling SUGGESTIONS

	WHITE SHIRT	SKINNY JEANS	HALTERNECK TOP	TUXEDO JACKET	BLACK WAISTCOAT	HIGH-WAISTED TROUSERS	SLINKY BLACK DRESS	ROCKER T-SHIRT	PLUNGE V-NECK SWEATER	*Now...* ACCESSORISE YOUR OUTFIT
1	✓	✓			✓					SKINNY TIE, BLACK POINTY BOOTS
2		✓	✓	✓						BLACK CLUTCH AND BLACK BOOTS
3	✓					✓				BLACK BALLET PUMPS, CHUNKY BANGLES
4		✓						✓	✓	STUDDED BELT, POINTY BOOTS, LEATHER CUFF
5							✓			BLACK HEELS, BLACK CLUTCH, LONG NECKLACES
6		✓			✓			✓		BLACK PUMPS, CHUNKY BANGLES
7				✓			✓			BLACK HEELS, MONOCHROME BANGLES
8			✓	✓		✓				POINTY BOOTS, LONG NECKLACE
9	✓	✓							✓	POINTY BOOTS, STUDDED BELT
10		✓		✓				✓		POINTY BOOTS, LEATHER CUFF

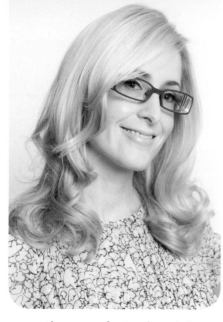

Wear it
YOUR WAY

AS ANY ROCKER KNOWS, RULES ARE MADE FOR BREAKING. This trend can be worn by all body shapes, but to guarantee the wow factor, here's how to make sure those bad-ass clothes complement your figure .

Pear Shapes
(carry weight on their hips and bum):

✦ Go for blazers/tuxedo jackets that fit and flare over the hips. This will highlight your slim upper body and make your bum look smaller.

✦ Instead of clingy dresses, try fitted shirts or tops with detail focused around the neck and shoulders that will stop the eye honing in on the hip area. Finish off by always wearing a low-slung belt to minimise lumps and bumps.

Apple Shapes
(carry weight on their tummy and chest):

✦ Never be tempted to wear anything clingy as this will only accentuate your rounded tummy. Instead opt for natural fabrics such as cotton that skim over the body and make sure tops are long enough to end on the hip.

- Wear skinny jeans and slim-leg trousers and tuck them into long pointed boots to really show off your pins.

Hourglass
(curvaceous all over with a small waist):

- Wear slightly cropped jackets but make sure lapels are wide enough to balance out your bust.
- Be careful about wearing strappy tops or halternecks. Even if you have the right bra on, spaghetti straps can make you look very top heavy. It might be classier to go for a top with wider straps so you can wear a more supportive bra.

Boy/Straight *(tall and lacking in curves):*

- All slim-fitting clothing will suit you, which gives you a big advantage. Go for narrow lapels, slim-line jackets and skinny jeans. Avoid wide belts as these will only accentuate your straightness. Instead go for skinny styles, or multiple belts which will help break up the torso.
- Go for empire-line tops that have a slight flare and come out from under the bust to help create the illusion of curves.

Strawberry Shaped
(broad shoulders and a wide back):

- Keep the focus on the bottom half of the body. Opt for flared skirts and trousers with a slight bootcut to help balance out your proportions. Don't wear halternecks or spaghetti straps; instead go for low-cut tops with sleeves to help soften bust. Wrap-around shirts are ideal.

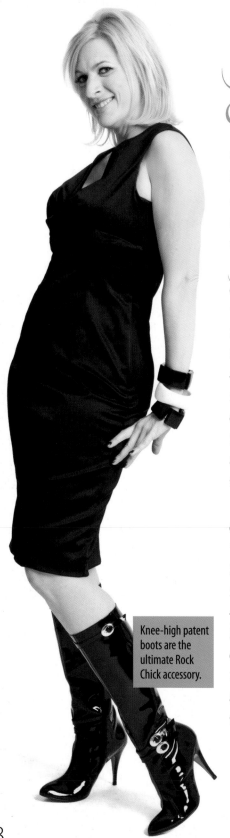

Knee-high patent boots are the ultimate Rock Chick accessory.

Seasoning

AS A TREND, ROCK CHICK LENDS ITSELF MORE TO A WINTER LOOK THAN A SUMMER WARDROBE, but there are small tweaks one can make to ensure wearability all year round.

Spring/Summer

1 LEGGINGS
2 OVERSIZED DARK SUNGLASSES
3 ANIMAL-PRINT HEADSCARF
4 JEWELLED OR METALLIC HEELED MULES
5 RED, WIDE-WAIST BELT
6 WHITE FITTED BLAZER
7 PALE-COLOURED PENCIL SKIRTS
8 METALLIC, BELTED TRENCH MAC
9 BIG GOLD CHAIN BELTS

Autumn/Winter

1 BERET
2 KNEE-HIGH, POINTED BOOTS
3 COLOURED OR FISHNET TIGHTS
4 COLOURED POLO NECKS
5 PATENT STILETTOS
6 BLACK, SEQUINED CAPE JACKET
7 STRUCTURED, PATENT LEATHER TOTE BAG
8 PATENT WIDE-WAIST BELT
9 BLACK TUXEDO SUIT

RECIPE FOR *Success*

THIS IS ONE TREND THAT REALLY EMBRACES YOUR INDIVIDUALITY AND SERVES AS A GREAT PLATFORM FOR EXUDING CONFIDENCE AND A VERY SASSY STYLE. The majority of your wardrobe is bound to be black, so play around with textures and fabrics to create different looks.

1. An Evening Event

A razor-sharp tux will look ultra glam for a drinks party. Go for black in winter and white in summer. Don't go too heavy with jewellery; opt for a large cocktail ring or a fine necklace as the focus should remain on the silhouette of the suit. Likewise don't overdo make-up; create smoky eyes and leave the rest bare.

2. The Weekend

Although this isn't the most practical look, a pared-down version can be great for a relaxing weekend. Wear skinny jeans with a white vest under a leather jacket, and accessorise with ballet pumps and a fierce studded belt.

3. A Date

To really send your date a-flutter, go for a slinky dress, accessorised with a low-slung chain belt and a large cuff or bangle, then choose between smoky, smouldering eyes or a kissable red pout.

4. Winter Time

Now your leather jacket will really come in handy – just make sure it doesn't have too much fringed and studded detail (far too Spinal Tap!). If you want something even warmer opt for a sharp tailored, black belted trench coat and wear with pointed black knee-length boots.

Make-Up Masterclass

ROCK CHICK MAKE-UP IS SULTRY, SEDUCTIVE AND EDGY – think Debbie Harry singing 'Heart of Glass' or Kate Moss with heavy, kohled eyes, neutral cheeks and lips and sexy bed-head hair. These expert make-up tips will give your look some serious edge.

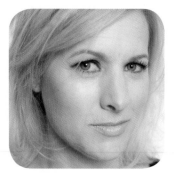

1. The Face

Illuminating your face can knock years off your complexion and will give tired, lacklustre skin the appearance of eight hours of blissful beauty sleep.

✦ Wear a sheer foundation close to your skin tone. Apply to your T-zone and blend outwards.

✦ Apply creamy concealer one shade lighter than your foundation under the eye and blend downwards and across into the top of your cheekbone.

✦ Set foundation and concealer using a yellow-based loose powder.

✦ Create points of light with an illuminating pen two shades lighter than your foundation. Apply to the area just below the eyebrows, the upper regions of your cheekbone, the space between the eyebrows, and in the hollow of your chin.

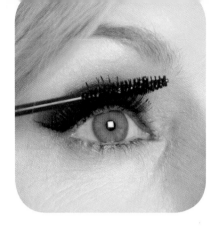

2. Smoky Eyes

Smoky eyes are a style staple for any fashionista regardless of their vintage. You will need a light, medium and dark shade of the same colour. I love smoky eyes in grey, plums, navy or browns, as they're kinder and more flattering as we get older.

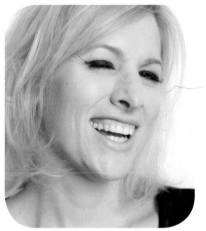

✦ Prep the eyelid. The key to keeping eyeshadow from melting into your eyelid crease as the day goes on is to keep eyelids oil-free. To do this start with an eyeshadow base.

✦ Apply the lightest colour from lash line to the crease of your eye. Press colour on instead of applying with brush strokes. This will produce a more intense effect and enables better control of colour.

✦ Press the medium colour shadow onto the crease. Then use a soft brush to blend and fade the edges of your shadows together.

✦ Take an angled eyeliner brush, dip it into water and work the brush into the darkest eyeshadow shade. Press the colour into the lash line, as close to the lashes as possible, both top and bottom. Your aim is to get a soft, smudged line rather than a solidly opaque one.

✦ Stroke on the blackest of black mascara to the top lashes. Really work the brush through your top lashes, then brush lightly through bottom lashes. Lastly, smudge the medium eyeshadow shade under the eye with a Q-tip.

Drop Dead Hair

ROCK CHICK HAIR IS SLIGHTLY UNRULY. The trick is to create a style that doesn't look overly groomed.

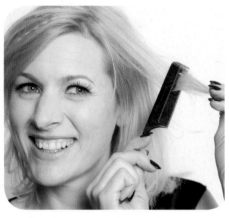

1. Bed Head

✦ Apply medium-hold style spray to the roots on towel-dried hair.

✦ Using a hairdryer, direct the heat at the roots and use your fingers to lift them. When roots are dry, take the heat through to the ends, styling with your fingers as you go. This creates a messy, un-done look.

✦ When dry, blast your hair upside down on a cool setting – do ing this will set your style.

✦ Finally tip your hair up, comb through and style using your fingers

2. The Middle Road

Give your hair an unstyled look by zigzagging the parting.

✦ Place the pointed tail of a comb at the front of your parting where you want the zigzag part to start.

✦ When you reach the end of where you want the zigzag part to end, place your forefinger close to the comb tail and pull both your hand and the comb down your head in the exact opposite direction.

✦ Continue the same way until you reach the back of your head.

Gorgeous
SINGING SENSATIONS

THE MUSIC INDUSTRY MAY STILL BE A MAN'S WORLD, but Madonna and Debbie Harry aren't the only sisters doing it for themselves. Let these sexy, ballsy female singers inspire you to find your inner Rock Chick.

1. *Gwen Stefani* – With her bindis, white blonde hair and bright red lips, the former No Doubt singer's got the looks to match her voice.

2. *Suzi Quatro* – Still looking fabulous at fifty-something, Suzi is the ultimate leather-clad rock 'n' roll icon.

3. *Beth Ditto* – Proving that Rock Chicks come in all shapes and sizes, The Gossip's lead singer is more than happy taking centre stage in neon brights, shiny leggings and vampy make-up.

4. *Courtney Love* – The epitome of wild child excess, Courtney looks fierce and feisty with her platinum blonde hair and pouty, come-to-bed lips.

5. *Alison Goldfrapp* – This twenty-first century Rock Chick ramps up the drama with vintage clothes, false eyelashes and wild stage costumes.

6. *Pink* – Toned to within an inch of her life, this bestselling singer looks tough and feminine in sexy, figure-hugging outfits. No wonder she always gets the party started!

7. *Chrissie Hynde* – Effortlessly cool in sharp, masculine tailoring, smoky eye make-up and her trademark heavy fringe, the lead singer of The Pretenders became the voice of her generation.

chapter 3

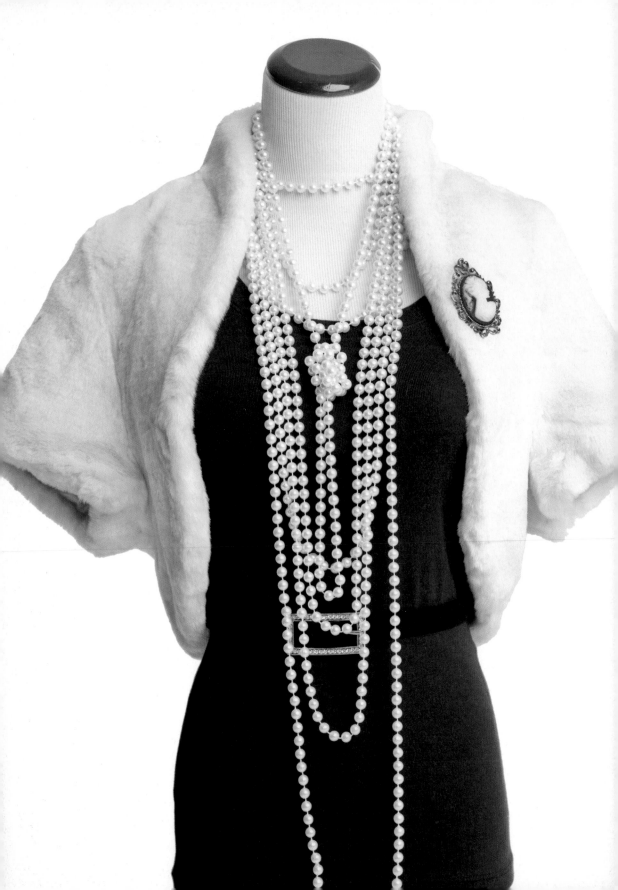

GROWN-UP
Glamour

BRING ON THE TWINSET AND PEARLS – IT'S
TIME TO LOOK PRIM AND ACT PROPER, IN
TRUE LADYLIKE FASHION OF COURSE!

'YOUR DRESSES SHOULD BE TIGHT ENOUGH TO SHOW YOU'RE A WOMAN AND LOOSE ENOUGH TO SHOW YOU'RE A LADY.'

Edith Head

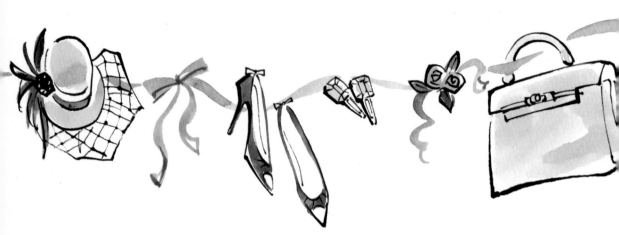

POST-WAR
Fashions

THIS LOOK IS INSPIRED BY THE STYLE OF THE LATE 1940S AND 50S AND IS ALL ABOUT SHOW-STOPPING GLAMOUR – immaculate clothes, pristine make-up and not a hair out of place – which makes it a style for anyone who wants to get noticed and look drop-dead gorgeous. The great thing about **Grown-Up Glamour** is that it looks amazing on women of all ages, and suits all shapes and sizes.

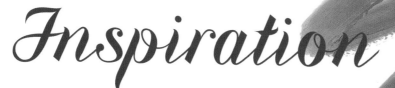

Inspiration
FROM THE A-LIST

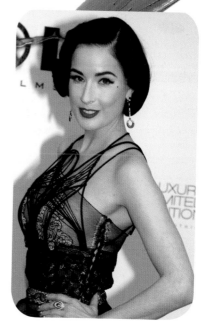

WITH HER PERFECT RED POUT, CINCHED-IN HOURGLASS FIGURE AND IMMACULATE COMPLEXION, the flawless **DITA VON TEESE** is the epitome of this look, inspiring fashionistas and top designers with her elegant take on old Hollywood mystique. As her popularity rose, the French couturiers began queuing up to adorn her body in figure-hugging gowns and flirtatious high heels. But Dita has stayed true to her own personal style, continuing to mix contemporary fashion with fabulous vintage finds. A lifelong fan of 1940s fashion, her carefully cultivated image marks her out as a complete individual, and it can hardly fail to inspire us all to give **Grown-Up Glamour** a whirl.

'I MIX VINTAGE WITH MODERN … I AM NOT AFRAID TO TAKE RISKS.'
Dita Von Teese

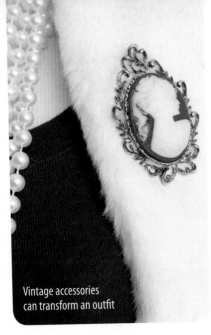

Vintage accessories
can transform an outfit

Gorgeous...
GLAMOROUS TREATS

WHEN YOU'RE RUSHED OFF YOUR FEET ALL DAY, IT CAN BE HARD
TO FIND A MOMENT FOR YOURSELF. But take the time to treat
yourself like the goddess you really are, and I guarantee that you'll
emerge feeling like a million dollars. Take a tip from Dita and co.,
and spoil yourself with these glamourous treats:

1. Manicure

Your mum was right: it's hard to be sophisticated with chipped varnish and
bitten-down nails, young lady!

2. Pedicure

Even if it's winter and you're hiding your feet inside socks and shoes every
day, it'll give you a boost to know your toes are looking picture-perfect.

3. Decadent Dinner Reservation

Whether you're raising the romantic stakes or treating a friend to a slap-up
meal, a trip to a fancy restaurant is the perfect excuse for dressing up and
letting loose.

4. Professional Blow-Out

Got a hot date or a scary interview? A salon-perfect do will make you feel like the world's at your (perfectly manicured) feet.

5. Silk Underwear

There' are few things guaranteed to put a spring in your step (and your man's too!) than knowing that underneath your everyday clothes is a gorgeous layer of luxury.

6. Exotic Bath Oils

If you've had a hard day, sometimes cheap bubble bath just won't cut it. Treat yourself to some fancy suds, lock the door and let your troubles float away.

7. Vintage Accessories

Whether its a silk scarf or a sparkly brooch, retro accessories are an inexpensive way to transform an outfit and make you feel frivolous and ultra-feminine.

8. Regular Facials

Whether you do it yourself or shell out for a spa, a monthly facial will keep your pores clear, your skin soft and your complexion sparkling whatever your age.

9. Designer Sunglasses

Channel your favourite Hollywood superstar by splurging on some dazzling A-list shades.

10. Posh Chocolates

This look is all about celebrating womanly curves, so give the diet a break for once. After all, nothing is sexier than a woman who indulges herself now and then!

Key INGREDIENTS

THE ULTRA-FEMININE STYLES OF THE 1940S AND 50S CONTINUE TO HAVE A STRONG INFLUENCE ON FASHION TRENDS TODAY. Full skirts, pencil skirts, pussy-bow blouses, and voluminous sleeves are all high street staples. Here are all the wardrobe essentials you'll need to give yourself a little retro glamour:

1 PENCIL SKIRT

For a sexy and flattering fit, choose one that is quite fitted. It shouldn't pull, but should be a slim fit around the thighs and taper in slightly towards the knees. In my experience most women can carry off a PENCIL SKIRT as long as they dress it with a pair of heels. Remember that curves are sexy! Too many of us cover up our bodies with loose, badly fitting clothes. Instead show off your curves in a figure-hugging skirt – you'll never look back!

> *Tip* *As a general rule, a SKIRT that sits on or just above the knee is much more flattering. If you really don't like your knees, find one that finishes just above your calf, creating the illusion of a slimmer thigh.*

2 FULL CIRCULAR SKIRT

Full voluminous SKIRTS have become extremely popular on the high street as they are so easy to wear and the added volume makes your legs look wonderfully slim. They nip in at the waist and cover a multitude of sins. More versatile than pencil skirts, they can be worn casually with ballet pumps, or dressed up with heels and a belt.

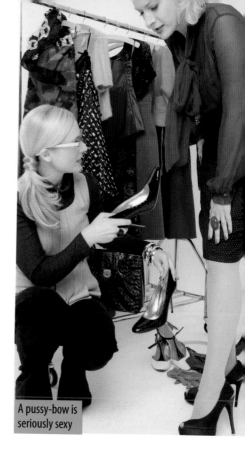

A pussy-bow is seriously sexy

3 PUSSY-BOW BLOUSE

The PUSSY-BOW BLOUSE is actually one of the most difficult elements of this look to get right. Get it wrong, and you'll look frumpy rather than fabulous. Get it right, and you'll look seriously sexy. If you're struggling, opt for a fitted knit top with a bow set at the very bottom of the V-neck.

4 BUSTIER

There is nothing better to shape a waistline or lift your cleavage, so don't just save your BUSTIER for best. Wear with a pair of jeans and heels for a sexy, understated look. Also a good corset can be inexpensive, so invest in a simple design and a radiant colour to really set off your complexion.

5 VOLUMINOUS SLEEVES

A godsend if you're worried about bingo wings, large VOLUMINOUS SLEEVES are soft, feminine and an ideal way to balance out the hips. When choosing a bell-shaped sleeve opt for soft, sheer fabrics like chiffon as they will drape better and flatter the arm.

6 BOXY JACKET

Inspired by the 1950s, these JACKETS flatter most figures, but their cropped style means they are particularly good on shorter women. Team with a pair of neat trousers or a straight skirt and heels for a slimming effect. Boxy jackets with ¾-length sleeves are particularly flattering as you'll be able to layer a long-sleeved top underneath – creating interest and adding definition to the arm.

7 PRINTED TEA DRESS

Flirty, sexy and fun, the TEA DRESS captures the timeless femininity of the '40s, evoking summer picnics in poppy-speckled fields or high tea on the green. They remain one of the most popular vintage buys, irrespective of catwalk trends. Spring is the time to hit the high street in search of these delicate dresses, made from layers of chiffon, printed with dots or gorgeous florals, and bound at the waist with a satin ribbon or slim belt.

> *Tip* *If you're lucky enough to find a VINTAGE DRESS, don't match with vintage shoes, but team with sharper, modern footwear for a more contemporary feel. You won't regret it.*

8 SLIM-LEG TROUSERS

SLIM-LEG TROUSERS are great if you've got the legs for them, but straight-leg are a better option for those with curvier figures. If you're trying out this look for the first time, invest in a black pair with a lot of stretch – they'll be comfortable to wear and flattering too.

9 BOLERO JACKET

Tricky to wear, as they're severely cropped and quite unforgiving. That said, BOLEROS are fantastic when you need a layer to cover your arms but don't want to detract from the outfit.

> *Tip* *BOLEROS are ideal for teaming with circular skirts where another jacket style would add bulk to an already voluminous look. Just keep everything underneath simple.*

10 STRAPLESS GOWN

The STRAPLESS FITTED EVENING DRESS is a popular choice on the red carpet as it's got guaranteed wow factor. For non-A-listers, the opportunities to wear such a dress are few and far between. However, opting for something shorter in length – as opposed to an evening gown – will make it more versatile while still having impact.

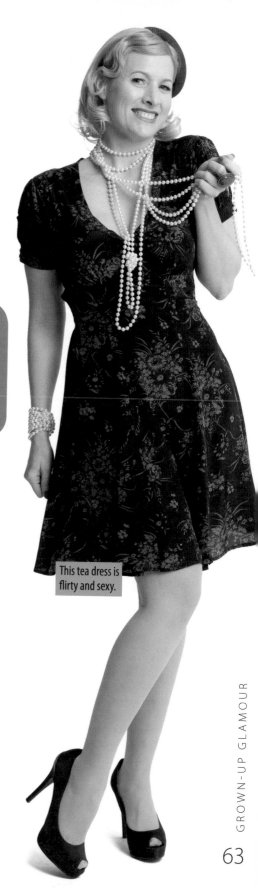

This tea dress is flirty and sexy.

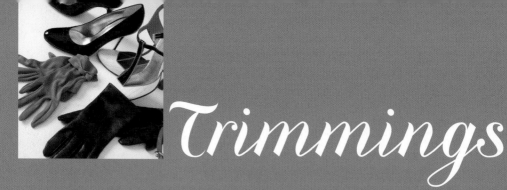

Trimmings

THIS LOOK IS ALL ABOUT GROOMING AND FINISHING TOUCHES. It's not enough to throw on a blouse and skirt - it's the right accessories that will turn you into a **Grown-Up Goddess**.

✦ FISHNET OR SEAMED TIGHTS

Perfect with a pencil skirt and heels for the ultimate sexy secretary look and an easy way to glam up your work clothes for the evening. When choosing FISHNETS, smaller nets are more flattering; or if you've got chunky carves, seamed tights are a chic, slimming option.

✦ KELLY BAG

With its smart tailored shape and timeless design, Grace Kelly's favourite HERMÈS BAG is one of the most iconic bags in history – and also one of the most expensive. Fortunately, there are plenty of copycat styles on the high street. Look for a metal-framed snap-clasp bag that's worn in the crook of the arm.

✦ BELT

Essential for creating that screen idol hourglass shape. Wide-waist BELTS are great at giving you curves, but a skinny belt is ideal when there's a lot of detail or a bold print on your outfit and you don't want your belt to compete with it.

✦ OPAQUE PATTERNED TIGHTS

If you're conscious of your legs, don't go for fishnets but try some stylish OPAQUE TIGHTS with a subtle pattern to create the same ladylike effect.

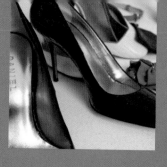
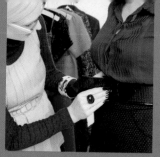
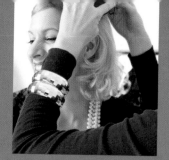

✦ CAMEO BROOCH

Potentially frumpy, but worn right, a BROOCH can bring a gorgeous vintage twist to a look. Wear as a choker, alongside other brooches on a jacket, or on a chain as a necklace for a more contemporary twist.

✦ STRAND OF PEARLS

Opt for large, chunky PEARLS or a few long strings worn together. You can also wrap around your wrist to create a cuff, or drape across hips or waist to create a beaded belt.

✦ LADYLIKE SCARF

SCARVES are a great accessory – wear them around the neck, as a belt, tied at the wrist, over a skirt, or around the strap of a handbag. As necklines are quite low with this style, fill in the space by wearing a neck scarf rakishly to the side.

✦ GLOVES

GLOVES are extremely elegant and also an ideal way of covering your hands if you feel they give your age away. My grandmother never went anywhere without a pair of gloves.

✦ POINTED COURT SHOE

For true glamour, it's heels all the way – the higher and pointier the better. POINTED COURT SHOES are flattering for most women and will elongate and slim your legs.

✦ T-BAR SHOE

T-BAR SHOES can be vamped up with a fancy buckle, lacing or a wide ankle strap, and they're wonderfully comfortable.

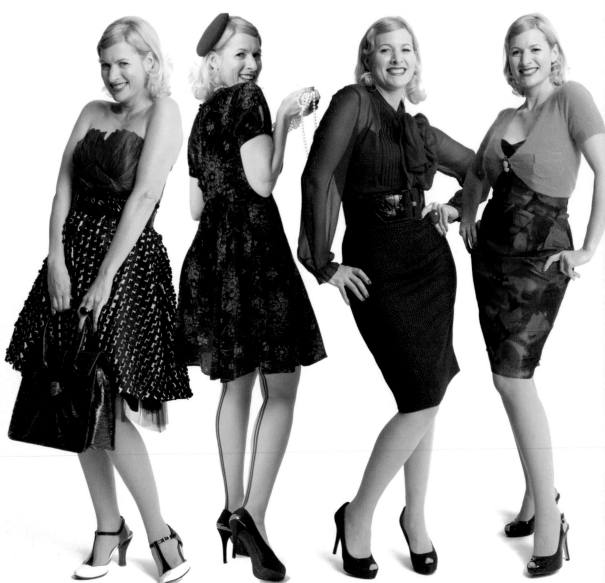

✦ The full circular skirt + bustier + T-bar shoes

✦ The flirty tea dress + pearls + seamed tights

✦ The pencil skirt + wide-waist belt + pussy-bow blouse

✦ The evening dress + bolero + cameo brooch

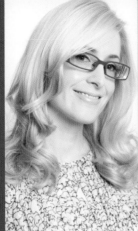

Styling SUGGESTIONS

	Pencil Skirt	Pussy-Bow Blouse	Full Skirt	Boxy Jacket	Printed Tea Dress	Slim-Leg Trousers	Bolero	Bustier	Evening Gown	Now... ACCESSORISE YOUR OUTFIT
1	✓	✓								WIDE-WAIST BELT, POINTED COURT SHOES, KELLY BAG AND FISHNET TIGHTS
2							✓		✓	CHANDELIER EARRINGS, AND LARGE COCKTAIL RING
3		✓		✓		✓				SLIM BELT, KELLY BAG AND T-BAR SHOES
4	✓			✓						SLIM WAIST-BELT, CAMEO BROOCH AND STRAND OF PEARLS
5		✓	✓							WIDE-WAIST BELT, POINTED COURT SHOES AND KELLY BAG
6	✓							✓		WIDE-WAIST BELT, STRAND OF PEARLS AND POINTED COURT SHOES
7			✓				✓			WIDE-WAIST BELT, LADYLIKE SCARF AND KELLY BAG
8						✓		✓		SLIM-WAIST BELT, LADYLIKE SCARF AND T-BAR SHOES
9					✓		✓			STRAND OF PEARLS, CAMEO BROOCH, POINTED COURT SHOES
10			✓	✓						FITTED T-SHIRT, LADYLIKE SCARF AND WIDE WAIST BELT

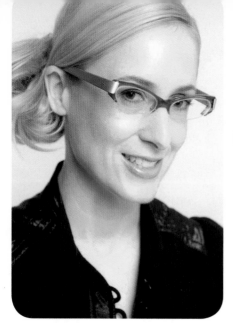

Wear it
YOUR WAY

MAKE SURE EVERYTHING YOU WEAR IS FITTED. There's a fine line between frumpy and sexy when it comes to **Grown-Up Glamour,** so flaunt your curves! The waist is the focal point for this look, but if you are not a natural hourglass there are certain tricks that can give the illusion of a balanced, curvaceous Old Hollywood figure:

Pear Shapes
(carry weight on their hips and bum):

✦   Choose tops that are fitted at the body and have volume on the sleeves. This will emphasise your slim waist.

✦   Avoid boxy shapes and opt for jackets that really cinch in at the waist and skim out over the hips. Make sure jackets finish at bottom of hips to ensure correct fit and proportion.

Apple Shapes
(carry weight on their tummy and chest):

✦   Opt for tea dresses with a full skirt that is tied loosely at the waist. Choose chiffon fabric that will skim over the body not cling.

✦   Avoid pencil skirts as these will only highlight the problem area. Instead go for a 50s circular skirt with a wide waistband that sits just

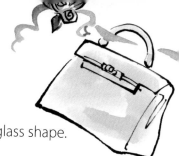

under the belly button – this will create an hourglass shape.

Hourglass
(curvaceous all over with a small waist):

✦ Go for fitted styles to flaunt your curves. Make a real feature of your waist by adding a wide belt in a contrasting colour to your outfit.

✦ Bustier tops can often make hourglasses with larger chests look top heavy. Team with a little bolero for ladylike modesty.

✦ Fitted and flared jackets look fantastic, but don't go for styles that button up too high.

Boy/Straight *(tall and lacking in curves):*

✦ Always opt for belts to create a waist but don't go too wide – a maximum width of two inches will ensure a more curved, girly look.

✦ Fuller skirts tend to swamp slender frames. Opt for a classic pencil skirt to show off your slimness.

Strawberry Shaped
(broad shoulders and a wide back):

✦ Avoid fussy high-necked blouses as they will draw attention to your broad shoulders. Instead go for low V-necks to draw the eye down the body.

✦ Go for pin-tuck details on the shoulders of tops to soften squareness but avoid too much volume in sleeves as this will only add width.

✦ Don't go for straight skirts – we're not after a tube effect! Instead go for full circular skirts and dresses to help give you perfect proportions.

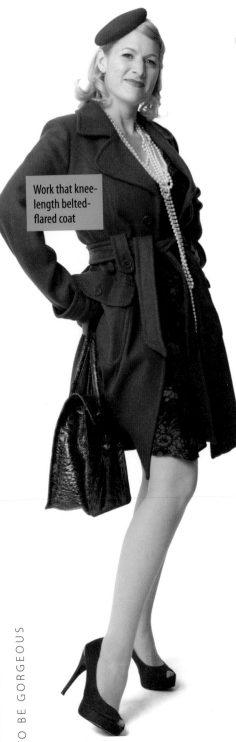

Work that knee-length belted-flared coat

Seasoning

THIS MAY NOT BE THE EASIEST LOOK IN THE BOOK, BUT IT'S CERTAINLY ONE YOU CAN RELY ON ALL YEAR ROUND, WHATEVER THE OCCASION. If you decide this is a style you really want to invest in, here are some seasonal basics to have you looking ladylike all through the year:

Spring/Summer

1 1950S HALTERNECK DRESS
2 SLEEVELESS FLARED SHIRTDRESS
3 PRETTY RUFFLE BLOUSE
4 HALTERNECK TOP
5 BELTED FLARED KNEE-LENGTH MAC
6 CAPRI PANTS
7 BALLET PUMPS
8 VINTAGE SILK WRAP

Autumn/Winter

1 KNEE-LENGTH BELTED FLARED COAT
2 TWEED SKIRT SUIT
3 WOOL PENCIL SKIRT
4 FAUX FUR STOLE
5 PILLBOX HAT
6 WOOLLEN CAPE
7 CHANDELIER EARRINGS
8 ELBOW-LENGTH GLOVES

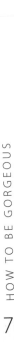

RECIPE FOR *Success*

ASK YOURSELF: WHAT WOULD **DITA** DO? Looking smartly groomed at all times isn't easy if you have a busy lifestyle, but there are still many occasions when you can have fun dressing up like a retro glamour girl.

1. The Office

Boxy skirt suits teamed with a fitted knit top or blouse are perfect if you're running in and out of meetings all day. Alternatively, a pencil skirt teamed with a pussy-bow blouse and neat little belt will take you from day to dinner with just a quick swish of lippy.

2. The Cocktail Party

For a formal drinks party where a little grown-up glitz is required, try a fitted knee-length evening dress, belted at the waist, with a strapless or low-cut neckline. A beautiful necklace and stiletto court heels will finish the look.

3. The Black-Tie Event

A long strapless, fishtail gown in a bold colour, with a choker or large chandelier earrings and a pretty beaded purse bag will give you real, old-style Hollywood glamour. If you're worried about your arms then just add a wrap or a bolero jacket.

4. The Wedding Outfit

For a summer wedding, a pretty tea dress with a subtle print can be gorgeous. Pick out one of the colours in the print to find shoes to complement and pull the look together, and add a structured clutch bag.

Make-Up Masterclass

THE GLAMOUR GIRLS OF THE 1940S AND 50S wouldn't have been seen dead stepping out of the house without flawless skin, a little flick of eyeliner and lashings of foxy red lipstick. The whole look is about looking polished and ultra-feminine, so emanate a classic beauty that will never date with my guide to glamorous grooming.

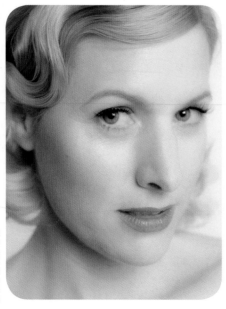

1. Michivieous Eyes

Eyes are kept relatively simple for this look, so as not to compete with your statement red lips, but they should still have a sexy, cheeky look. Eyebrows are heavy and arched and eyeliner 'ticks' up at the outer corner of the eyes. This easy-to-achieve eye make-up screams retro sex kitten.

✦ Keep your eyebrows a natural thickness, but have them shaped into clean, well-defined arches.

✦ Accentuate their shape by using a

brow pencil to fill in any gaps. Apply the eyebrow pencil in short feathered strokes to mimic your natural brows.

✦ Set into shape with a clear mascara or a little hair wax.

✦ Sweep a bone-coloured eyeshadow over your entire eyelid.

✦ Use a highlighting eye pencil just under the arch of your eyebrow to further enhance the shape of your arch.

✦ Using a black liquid eyeliner carefully create a little tick at the outer corners of both eyes as close to the lash line as possible.

✦ Apply mascara to your top and lower lashes.

2. A Perfect Shade of Red

A scarlet pout oozes femininity and confidence, but it's very important to find a shade that suits you. Here's how to turn heads by finding your perfect red:

✦ The most important thing to consider when choosing a red lipstick is your skin tone.

✦ If you have WARM, yellow tones, you will best suit a red with a golden, tawny or orange base.

✦ If you have COOL, pink tones to your skin, go for lipsticks that have blue undertones.

✦ For ASIAN skin, berry tone reds are perfect.

✦ Don't test the lipstick colour on the back of your hand. Instead, always apply the lipstick with a clean lip brush to your lips and walk into daylight to check the shade against your skin tone.

✦ Don't be tempted to match your lipstick to whatever handbag, necklace or shoes you may be wearing. A different but complementary shade of red will look much more modern.

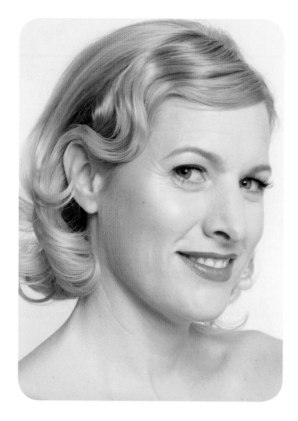

Drop Dead Hair

1. The Posh Ponytail

If you're feeling more prim than pin-up, go for a preppy 50s look with a straight, sleek ponytail and a heavy fringe.

✦   Blow-dry hair straight, and then lightly backcomb to inject volume.

✦   Brush hair back into a ponytail with a paddle brush and secure with a hair band.

✦   Take a long strand of hair from underneath the ponytail and spray heavily with hairspray until stiff. Wrap around the base of the ponytail to conceal the hair band. Fix in place with a slim-line grip.

✦   Tame flyaway hair with a spritz of hairspray, and for added polish, run a shine serum through your ponytail and fringe.

1. Pin-Up Curls

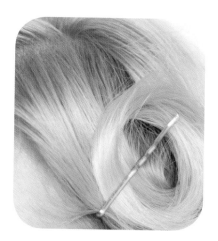

Many of the world's hottest celebrities are sporting hairstyles that are reminiscent of retro Hollywood glamour girls. However, you don't need a personal stylist to make like Marilyn Monroe with these tried-and-tested tips for perfect pin curls.

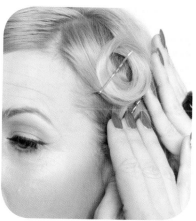

✦ Get your hair about 80% dry, then comb a curl-setting lotion through to the ends of the hair.

✦ Next, take small sections of hair, curl them tightly around a hot tong, hold in place for a few moments and then release. Make sure you secure the ends to avoid frizzing.

✦ Wrap the curl around your finger and use a hair grip to fasten to your head.

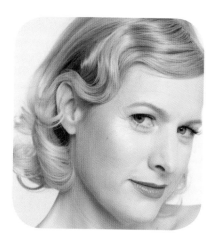

✦ When you have finished curling your entire head, remove the grips and run a smoothing lotion through your hair with your fingers. Do not brush.

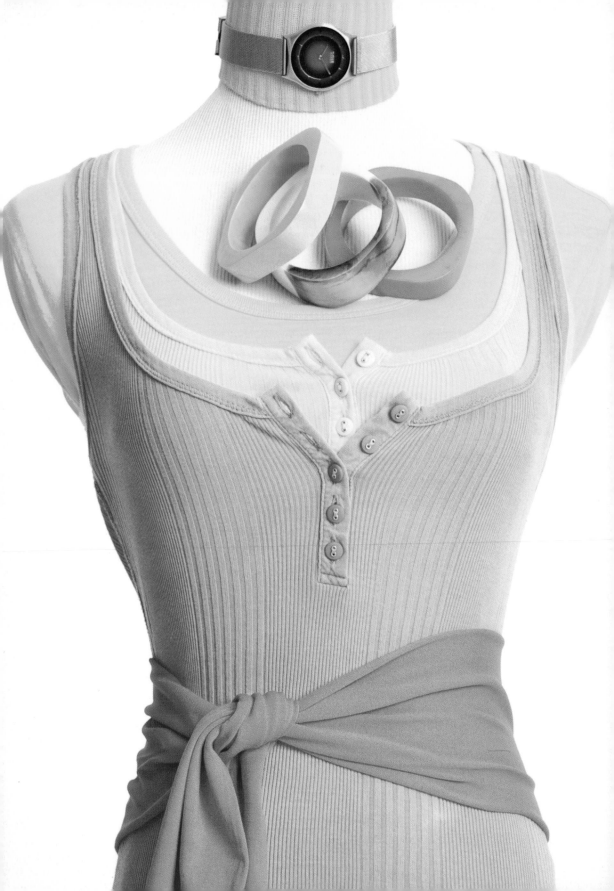

chapter 4

SPORTS *Luxe*

YOU DON'T HAVE TO LOVE LYCRA TO APPRECIATE
THIS SEXY, URBAN STYLE. GIVE IT A CHANCE, AND
YOU'LL SEE THAT SPORTS LUXE CAN BE A LOOK
THAT WILL GET YOUR HEART PUMPING.

'I HAVE ALWAYS BEEN INTO WEARING WHAT I LIKE, FOR ME CLOTHES NEED TO BE COMFORTABLE, I HATE BEING RESTRICTED.'
Cameron Diaz

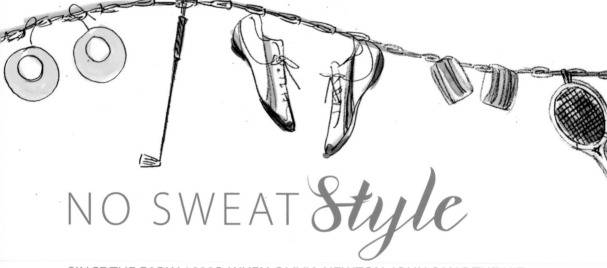

NO SWEAT *Style*

SINCE THE EARLY 1980S, WHEN OLIVIA NEWTON-JOHN SANG THE HIT SINGLE 'LET'S GET PHYISCAL', active wear has moved out of the gym and into the spotlight and begun to set new style records.

Performance fabrics such as parachute cloth, spandex and fleece that were once reserved for actual sporting activities have been redesigned into modern, everyday clothing, which combine practicality with a fresh utilitarian style. Sports Luxe is all about making it easy for women to look stylish without breaking into a sweat.

Inspiration
FROM THE A-LIST

BEST KNOWN FOR HER RELAXED SURFER STYLE, CAMERON DIAZ's offbeat dress sense is all about balance and simplicity. Always seen in simple clean lines, she uses bold colours to work the casual urban look. Cameron's sporty style involves a refreshing 'less is more' attitude towards fashion, that means her wardrobe staples are colourful fitted T-shirts, skinny jeans and comfortable, super-flattering jersey dresses.

By contrast JENNIFER LOPEZ is renowned for her urban street look, and she loves nothing better than throwing on brightly coloured **SPORTS LUXE** layers over tight slogan vest tops, then adding plenty of bling. By mixing and matching luxurious and functional fabrics, Jennifer has paved the way for women all over the world to emulate her sexy, laid-back style.

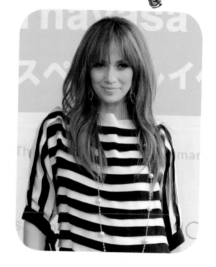

'MY FASHION SENSE IS EVER-EVOLVING. I LOVE WHEN GLAMOUR IS MIXED WITH A MODERN FEEL TO KEEP THE STYLE FRESH.'
Jennifer Lopez

Key INGREDIENTS

GET ANY THOUGHTS OF BAGGY TRACKSUITS OUT OF YOUR HEAD, this cool, urban look is flattering and versatile. You don't have to be Venus Williams to score an ace in these hardworking essentials.

1 METALLIC VEST TOP

Metallic fabrics look great when teamed with jeans or black trousers, since they reflect the light, disguise lumps and bumps, and add an element of futuristic glamour.

2 BRIGHT RACER-BACK VEST

These tops with the cut-out backs can be layered over each other or over straight-backed vests and T-shirts to add a colourful, sporty twist to your outfit.

> *Tip* If you're conscious about your T-SHIRT riding up, buy a top one size up to layer underneath your regular size. This will give you extra coverage while making it easier to see the layers.

3 RUGBY/POLO SHIRTS

Think Catherine Zeta-Jones looking fresh and flirty on the golf course. The important thing is to go for a shirt that's fitted and brightly coloured, not shapeless and dingy. **RUGBY SHIRTS** traditionally have collars, making them perfect for women with generous chests.

4 JEWEL-COLOURED SATIN TOP

This look is all about colour, fabric and shine, and you don't get more glamorous than **JEWEL-COLOURED SATIN**. Wear with jeans, or tucked into a skirt, this top is a worthwhile investment that'll add glitz to any outfit.

Tip Don't overdo the satin or shine. Make the top the focus and team with muted colours and minimal accessories to avoid looking OTT.

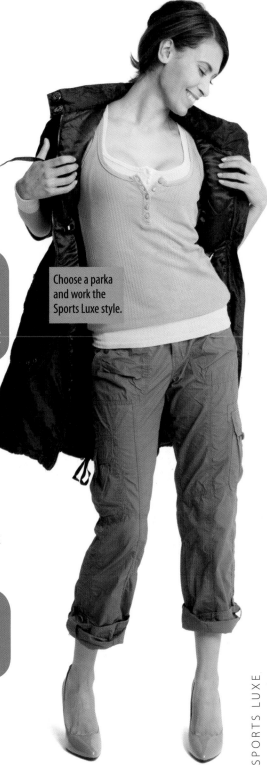

Choose a parka and work the Sports Luxe style.

5 PARKA COAT

The **PARKA** is a must-have for this look – easy to wear and ideal for the UK climate – but don't stick with plain black. Why not dare to be different and try one in a metallic finish? It'll be far more versatile, and you can work it day and night.

Tip There is a tendency to wear PARKAS open and slouchy. Choose one that's got shape in the waist.

SPORTS LUXE

81

6 HOODED TOPS

The word 'hoodie' immediately conjures up images of teenage boys hanging around the less salubrious parts of town. But the **HOODIE** can also be a classic element of a sporty, casual look. For maximum style and minimum ASBO connotations opt for a zip top that's fitted in the waist and team with a colourful vest and yoga-style pants or jeans.

7 PARACHUTE DRESS

This is the perfect solution for a hot day in the sun: an easy-to-wear **DRESS** that's slightly nipped in at the waist with plenty of volume at the bottom. This is a look that can be dressed down with designer trainers or pumps or spruced up with a pair of heels depending on whether you're shopping around town or off to a garden party.

> *Tip For ultra-slimming and body-skimming effect go for a DRESS in cotton or a fine jersey. To make it work in the winter, layer over long-sleeved T-shirts and leggings.*

8 JERSEY T-SHIRT DRESS

What you're after is a stretch-knit dress, either plain or with a large graphic or pattern emblazoned over it. This is a piece that's quite difficult to wear on its own unless you have a figure to die for. A more practical solution for the rest of us would be to layer the **T-SHIRT DRESS** over jeans or add a cropped bomber jacket to create a slimmer silhouette. If you go for a solid block of colour don't forget to accessorise with a long string of beads, chunky bracelets and a hipster belt for a more edgy look.

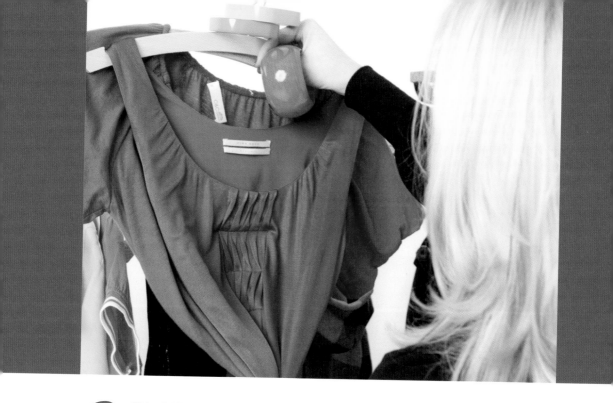

9 FLAT-FRONTED TROUSERS

Flat-fronted trousers are a great wardrobe basic as they can be dressed up (Jennifer Aniston style) with a blazer and pumps, or down (Cameron Diaz style) with Converse trainers and a T-shirt.

 Although black is a wardrobe staple, other muted colours such as charcoal, navy and soft grey are useful extras for working with bright, sporty colours.

10 PLEATED GYM-STYLE SKIRT

The beauty of this style SKIRT, is that it flatters most body shapes, as long as it's not too short — just above the knee is ideal. Wear with polo shirts or simple T-shirts layered under hooded tops, or make it more summery with a racer-back vest and designer trainers.

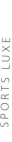

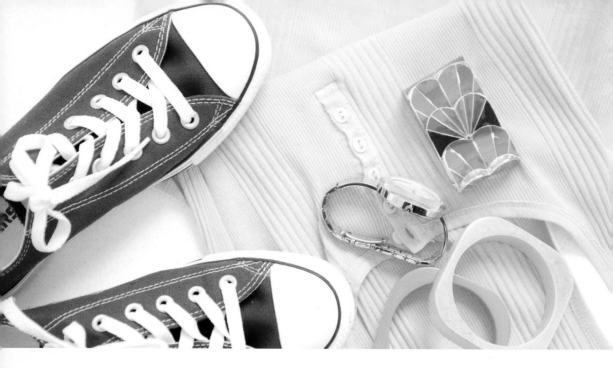

Trimmings

As this is a sporty, urban style, accessories are less obvious than in other looks. However, these few essentials will give you a winning edge.

✦ BIG WATCH

The sporty WATCH is a key accessory for this look. The bigger and the more functionality it has, the better, even if you don't know how to use it!

✦ SWEAT BANDS

If you really want to embrace this look, add a little tongue-in-cheek fun with kitschy SWEAT BANDS.

✦ LARGE BRIGHTLY COLOURED CUFF

This is a more workable alternative to the sweatband. Keeping it big and bold is important – fluorescent tones are popular with this trend.

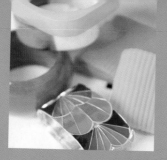
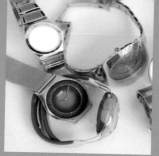
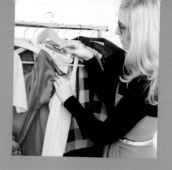

✦ METALLIC COURT SHOES

Choose pointy HEELS to elongate the leg and team with leggings or skinny jeans.

✦ DAYGLO BANGLES

Stack them together for an easy way to incorporate a flash of fluorescent without looking like a strobe light.

✦ SILVER HOOP EARRINGS

These are very sporty, and youthful, but be careful not to go too big as they may look cheap.

✦ DESIGNER TRAINERS

Don't be tempted to wear the same TRAINERS you wear to the gym with your day look. Designer trainers offer the comfort of a trainer without looking like a sport's shoe – making them more versatile.

✦ CONVERSE TRAINERS

CONVERSE TRAINERS have been a key element of the sport chic look for many years. Not only are they cool, but they're practical and unlikely to date.

✦ TENNIS SHOES

Your classic white TENNIS SHOE – as seen in the movie *Grease* – has made a comeback on the fashion front. These look great fresh out of the box, but it's tough to keep them in pristine condition.

✦ LARGE HOLDALL

A practical fashion essential for any busy mum. Try a large quilted version to keep it looking Luxe as well as sporty.

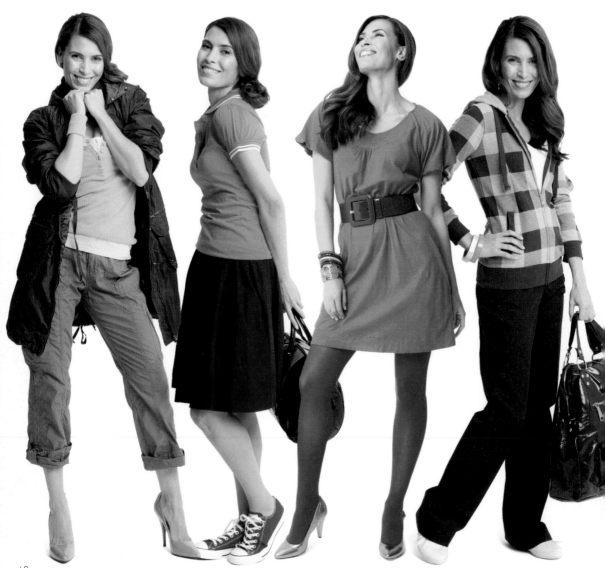

✦ The parka +
racer-back vest +
high-heeled courts

✦ The polo shirt
+ gym skirt +
Converse trainers

✦ The jersey T-shirt
dress + metallic
high-heeled courts

✦ The flat-fronted
trousers + hooded
top + tennis shoes

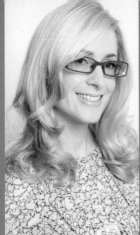

Styling
SUGGESTIONS

	METALLIC VEST	POLO SHIRT	SATIN TOP	PARKA	HOODED TOP	PARACHUTE DRESS	T-SHIRT DRESS	FLAT-FRONTED TROUSERS	RACER-BACK VEST	GYM SKIRT	Now... ACCESSORISE YOUR OUTFIT
1	✓			✓				✓			METALLIC HEELS, BIG WATCH, LONG BEADED NECKLACE
2		✓							✓		CONVERSE OR TENNIS SHOES
3	✓						✓				CONVERSE OR TENNIS SHOES, BANGLES
4						✓			✓		METALLIC HEELS, SILVER HOOP EARRINGS, CUFF
5					✓		✓				CONVERSE TRAINERS
6	✓			✓						✓	TENNIS SHOES, BIG WATCH
7			✓					✓			METALLIC HIGH HEELS, DENIM JACKET
8	✓				✓			✓			DESIGNER TRAINERS, BIG HOLDALL
9		✓								✓	TENNIS SHOES
10									✓	✓	CONVERSE, BRIGHT FITTED CARDIGAN OR DENIM JACKET

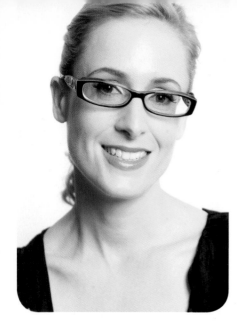

Wear it
YOUR WAY

THIS LOOK'S IDEAL FOR THE 'YUMMY MUMMY' WHO WANTS TO LOOK FASHIONABLE BUT STILL FEEL COMFORTABLE IN HER CLOTHES. Whether you're doing a marathon or the school-run, here's my guide to scoring high with the SPORTS LUXE look:

Pear Shapes
(carry weight on their hips and bum):

✦ Always layer vests to create more interest and give the illusion of wide, sporty shoulders.

✦ Stitch over side pockets on flat-fronted trousers as these tend to bulge, adding extra weight to the hips.

✦ Don't live in trainers! High, pointed court shoes will add length to your legs, slimming down your proportions.

Apple Shapes
(carry weight on their tummy and chest):

✦ Make sure that the fabric in your jersey dress is double-layered to stop it from clinging to your stomach.

✦ Avoid polo shirts with horizontal stripes – instead opt for plain colours.

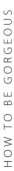

- Long-line jewel-coloured satin tops worn with a parka and skinny jeans will look gorgeous on you.

Hourglass
(curvaceous all over with a small waist):

- Go for short hoodies with deep waistbands to really emphasise your curves.
- With a polo shirt, always wear with the buttons open to avoid looking top-heavy.
- Halterneck parachute dresses will be particularly flattering as they give good cleavage, nip in the waist and disguise the hips.

Boy/Straight *(tall and lacking in curves):*

- Avoid big parachute skirts and go for pleated styles instead to create the illusion of a more curvy shape. Wear with fitted vest tops.
- Pull the drawstring of your jacket or parka tight to give yourself a shapely waist.
- Loose T-shirt dresses will suit your straight torso. Layer over skinny jeans and leggings to disguise skinny pins.

Strawberry Shaped
(broad shoulders and a wide back):

- Wear jewel-coloured satin tops that have a wide slash neck to soften the shoulders, or find designs that have a low V-neck opening.
- Don't layer vests as this will only add bulk – just stick with one at a time in a bold colour and team with a casual cardigan or hooded top.

Seasoning

THIS LOOK IS PRETTY STATIC THROUGHOUT THE SEASONS, making it very versatile and cost-effective to invest in. For die-hard SPORTS LUXE fans, here are a few seasonal additions you can add to your wardrobe to take your look to the next level.

Spring/Summer

1 NEON SUNGLASSES
2 VISOR
3 BRIGHT-COLOURED HIP-LENGTH RAINCOAT
4 MUTED KNEE-LENGTH SHORTS
5 SURFER BIKINI
6 RUBBER FLIP-FLOPS
7 WIDE BOY-CUT LINEN TROUSERS
8 FITTED, WASHED-OUT DENIM JACKET

Autumn/Winter

1 CROPPED BOMBER JACKET
2 BRIGHT OPAQUE TIGHTS
3 BLACK SLIM-LEG TROUSERS
4 COMBAT TROUSERS
5 SKINNY JEANS
6 LEGGINGS
7 NEON, POINTED COURT SHOES

Bright opaque tights look fabulous with jersey dresses.

RECIPE FOR *Success*

WITH THE MIX OF FABRICS AND BRIGHT COLOURS, THIS LOOK IS FIERCE ENOUGH FOR EVENING, but toned down and worn in the right way it can also give regular daywear a run for its money. Try it for:

1. *The Nightclub*

If you love to hit the dance floor every once in a while, why not team a jewel-coloured satin top with skinny jeans and bright heels? Don't forget a metallic parka to keep you warm on the way home, and an oversized clutch bag to dance around!

2. *After-Work Drinks*

For a fresh, Friday night look that'll take you all the way from work to last orders, wear a top with a drawstring bottom or press studs, a parachute skirt and your favourite heels.

3. *Weekend*

Even if you have nothing more energetic planned than pottering about and catching up with friends, why not try a cool hooded jacket with colourful vest underneath and a pair of skinny jeans. Go for trainers or heels depending on how long your legs are.

4. *Shopping*

For a smart casual take on this style, layer a dark jersey dress over a colourful T-shirt. Wear with tights and black heels in the winter or with bare legs and simple white tennis shoes when the sun comes out.

Make-Up Masterclass

DITCH HIGH-MAINTENANCE HAIR AND MAKE-UP in favour of a natural, sporty look. Look fresh-faced in a flash.

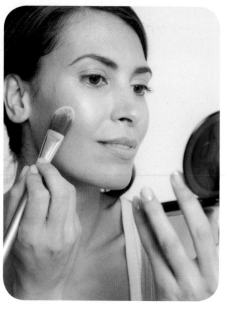

1. Good Foundations

The key to natural-looking make-up is choosing the right foundation for the job:

✦ Fine lines and wrinkles? Use mineral foundation for a smooth, youthful appearance.

✦ If your skin tends to be lacklustre try dewy finish foundation to give yourself a healthy glow.

✦ Outdoorsy? Tinted Moisturiser is perfect for a barely-there look that doubles up as a sunscreen.

✦ If your skin gets oily or spotty, go for either a liquid foundation that dries to a matte finish or a pressed powder foundation, and stay shine-free.

- Shop for foundation in daylight hours, not after dark.
- Don't assume that once you've found a good foundation, that's it for life. Our complexion changes as we get older and so you will need to change the foundation you use if you want to achieve a flawless finish.

2. Make Your Eye Colour Pop!

Cameron loves to play up the colour of her eyes and always opts for a shade that enhances the vivid colour of her irises. Here are some easy tips to help you choose your perfect eye colour . . .

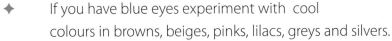

- If you have blue eyes experiment with cool colours in browns, beiges, pinks, lilacs, greys and silvers.
- For brown, hazel or green eyes try warmer colours such as purples, apricots, warm pinks, bronzes and golds.
- Select your preferred colour in a crème base formulation and pat onto your eyelids with your ring finger.
- Complete the look with a sweep of curling mascara to give eyes flirty lashes – a quick-fix alternative to using an eyelash curler.

3. Blush and Go

- Use a nude-coloured lipstick as cheek rouge! This is a great make-up artist trick which works brilliantly for an on-the-go SPORTS LUXE look, giving you that fresh 'just worked out' complexion.

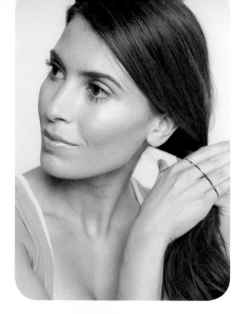

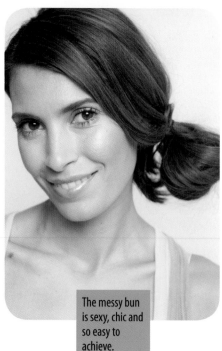

The messy bun is sexy, chic and so easy to achieve.

Drop Dead Hair

CAMERON DIAZ IS A PERFECT EXAMPLE OF A GIRL who always manages to make her hair look effortlessly sexy, in a 'just done in five minutes' kind of way, which works perfectly with her SPORTS LUXE style. Here's what to do if you want Cameron's sporty, slick look.

1. The Messy Bun

Today's hair bun is a far cry from the prim and proper librarian look of yesteryear. Instead, chic messy buns are all the rage. Not only are they easy to create, but they are incredibly versatile. You can wear them low in a classic chignon style or high on the head in the ballerina style and even to the side!

- Begin with clean, dry hair. Run a brush through it to smooth any tangles and apply an anti-frizz serum or gel.
- Brush your hair back into a ponytail. For a low bun secure the ponytail at the nape of your neck. For a higher bun secure the ponytail higher on the back of your head. Wrap the ponytail around its base and secure with second elastic on the back of your head, then secure the sides of the bun with bobby pins, tucking them into the back of the bun to pull it closer to your head.
- Pull out some small strands of hair with your fingers or a fine-tooth comb to give a slightly messy look.
- Spray the bun lightly with hairspray, to help it keep its shape.

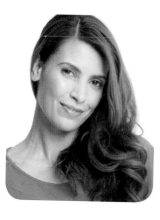

2. The Shaggy-Delic

Meg Ryan first made the shaggy hairstyle famous back in the 90s, and this style is now more popular than ever. Celebrities like Kate Moss and Sienna Miller all opt for this low-maintenance look. It's a great style for SPORTS LUXE since it doesn't require a lot of effort and it's fairly simple to achieve.

- Blow dry hair until it's 80% dry.
- Divide hair into six or eight sections and twist away from the face. Secure the twists with a clip and spray hair with a hairspray.
- Let hair dry the last 20% of the way.
- Take out the clips, flip your head over, and shake out the twists.
- Now flip your hair up and finger-comb apart. You'll notice little ridges in your hair. This creates a sexy just-out-of-bed, low-maintenance look.

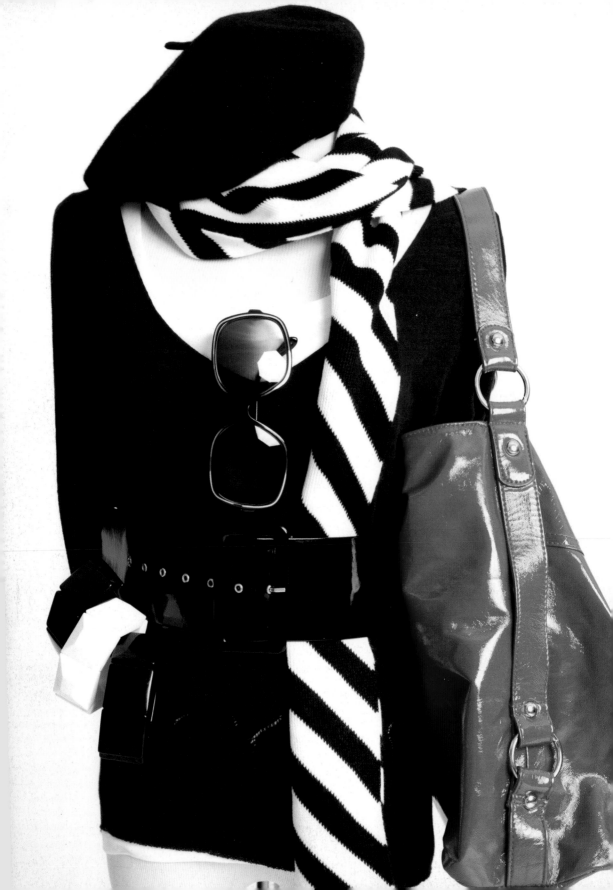

chapter 5

BREAKFAST AT

Tiffany's

IF YOU REALLY WANT TO SPARKLE, THIS
SOPHISTICATED BEATNIK STYLE IS QUITE SIMPLY
A GIRL'S BEST FRIEND.

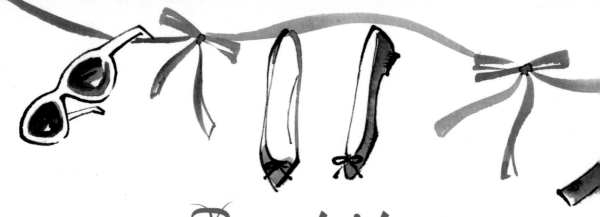

JUST *Beat it*

SOMETIMES FASHION CAN BE VERY BLACK AND WHITE . . . QUITE LITERALLY IN THE CASE OF THIS LOOK. Beatnik style consists of sharp, simple monochrome pieces worn together in a refreshingly uncluttered way – think Paris or New York in the 1950s and 60s.

Go girlish and gamine in a shift dress and ballet pumps, or Left Bank preppy in a black turtle-neck sweater and pedal-pushers, but make sure you remember the Hollywood shades to hide behind! Clean and chic, this is the perfect look for those aspiring to raise their style stakes.

Inspiration FROM THE A-LIST

IN 1957 AUDREY HEPBURN SANG AND DANCED HER WAY TO PARIS IN CLASSIC CULT MOVIE *FUNNY FACE*. As Jo Stockton, an intellectual bookshop clerk from Manhattan desperate to study philosophy on the Left Bank, Hepburn finds herself paying her way by reluctantly posing as a

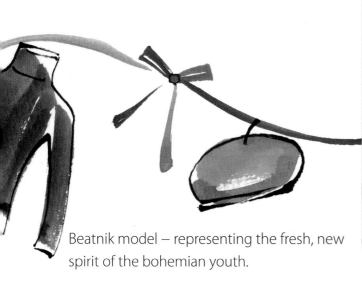

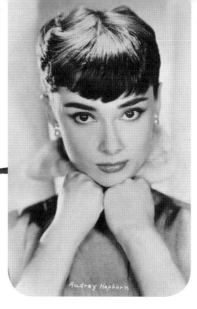

Beatnik model – representing the fresh, new spirit of the bohemian youth.

Hepburn spends the film being beautiful and intelligent in cool, understated clothing, so the Beatnik fashion really is a perfect fit. *Funny Face*'s monochrome style also became Hepburn's own uniform, making her the legendary style icon that she is today.

In her crisp white shirts, skinny polo necks and ballet pumps as flat as her chest, elegant Audrey was the complete opposite of her curvaceous contemporaries like Marilyn Monroe or Elizabeth Taylor. By 50s standards, she was too tall and too skinny, but rather than creating false curves, she chose clothes that accentuated her slenderness. With her boyish body, pixie haircut and swan neck she showed that women could dress androgynously yet still maintain their elegance and beauty.

'MY LOOK IS ATTAINABLE. WOMEN CAN LOOK LIKE AUDREY HEPBURN BY FLIPPING OUT THEIR HAIR, BUYING LARGE SUNGLASSES, AND A LITTLE SLEEVELESS DRESS.'

Audrey Hepburn

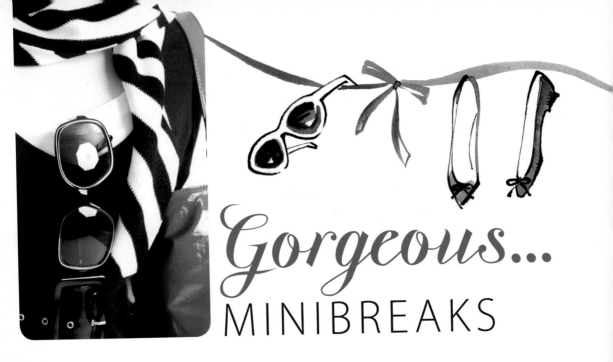

Gorgeous...
MINIBREAKS

AUDREY HEPBURN'S MOST ICONIC CHARACTERS PLAY OUT THEIR ROMANTIC DRAMAS AGAINST A BACKDROP OF THE WORLD'S MOST GORGEOUS CITYSCAPES. Why not follow suit, and indulge your inner superstar, with my top five stylish sojourns that won't break the bank.

Paris

The capital of romance and refined elegance. Parisians are known the world over for their classic chic. Be inspired by Audrey and pack your *slim-leg trousers*, *white T*, *black blazer* and some pretty *ballerina pumps*. Carry your maps and make-up in a stylish *tote*.

Rome

A city steeped in so much breathtaking architecture requires a pared-down glamour. Smart 50s-style *sundresses* teamed with fitted *cardigans* and *Mary-Janes* will help you take in the sights while blending in with the locals. Accessorise with a neat *shoulder bag* – Italian leather of course.

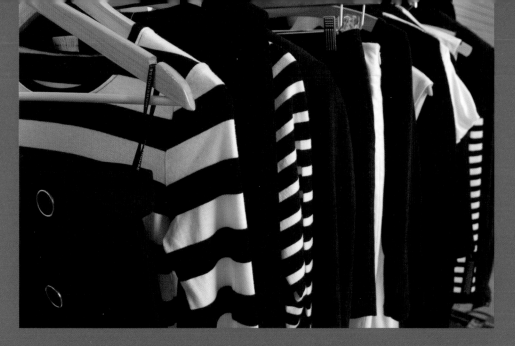

Barcelona

A *crisp shirt* worn with smart indigo *jeans* and Audrey's favourite *espadrilles* is a perfect combination for viewing Picasso's masterpieces. Pack your swimsuit into a *straw bag* and hit the beach after a hectic day in the galleries.

Marrakesh

For a heady treasure hunt around the labyrinth of Medinas, channel Audrey's evening look, with vibrant *printed maxi dresses* worn with *gladiator sandals*. Carry home your handmade trinkets in authentic ethnic *fabric bags*.

New York City

A stroll through Central Park, a trip up the Empire State building … even a little window-shopping at Tiffany's: in the Big Apple you'll feel like you're walking through a real-life movie set, so shine in traditional Audrey style: a simple *shift dress* reworked with *wedges* and *statement necklace* to see you through from day to night.

Key INGREDIENTS

THE BEAUTY OF THIS LOOK IS IN ITS SIMPLICITY. The elements are wardrobe staples that are worth investing in and will tide you over no matter what your age or size. Incorporate this style into your repertoire, and you'll never be at a loss for a timeless, elegant look.

1 CLASSIC WHITE SHIRT
Need I say more? We should all invest in at least one fitted, crisp **WHITE SHIRT**. Buy a couple to ensure they maintain their freshness.

2 SLIM-LEG BLACK TROUSERS/JEANS
If you're a true follower of this look, then **SLIM-FIT TROUSERS** and jeans are an essential buy. However, for those of us with larger legs, bootleg or straight-leg styles are a good alternative.

> *Tip* With all the elements in this look, quality is key. Invest in a good quality pair of TROUSERS that will hold their shape and colour for a chic, timeless look.

3 BLACK KNITTED DRESS
A simple **KNITTED SHIFT DRESS** or tunic is another Beatnik essential. Make sure the knit is of a good quality for a more flattering shape,

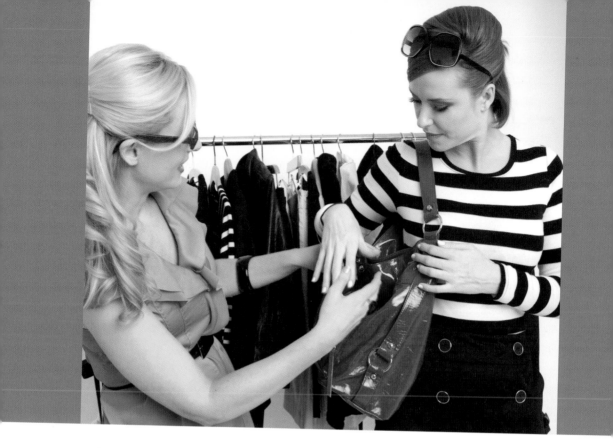

and don't be tempted to take it too short. To give you the confidence to wear a dress like this, you need good, supportive underwear that will give you a smooth finish.

4 BLACK AND WHITE STRIPED JUMPER

This is one of the few statement pieces in this look. **BLACK AND WHITE STRIPES** help to break up the starkness of this look without detracting from its Gallic simplicity. Wear over a white shirt with cuffs folded back over the jumper, or underneath a cropped black cape.

> *Tip* *Avoid wearing bold horizontal STRIPES if you've got a full chest; opt for stripes on accessories like scarves and shoes instead.*

5 BLACK POLO NECK

Another staple worth investing in, and once again quality is important. Useful for wearing under jackets or simply on its own with chic black trousers and pumps.

> *Tip* *Avoid POLO NECKS if you've got broad shoulders and a large chest as they'll square off your shape. Opt instead for a black V-neck sweater or knit wrap-around top. Polo necks also draw attention to your jaw line – so if you feel self-conscious about your chin, avoid!*

6 BLACK A-LINE SKIRT

Ideal for women of different ages and body shapes, the **BLACK A-LINE SKIRT** will be a versatile addition to your wardrobe. Team with white shirt and skinny belt or black polo neck, patterned tights and pumps.

7 FITTED BLACK BLAZER

Again, this is an item worth spending money on as it will last you for years to come; layer over a white shirt or striped jumper and team with jeans or trousers for a timeless look. Make sure it's fitted in the waist as this helps to create an hourglass shape, and remember that Beatnik black is very black. Consider re-dying blazers that are starting to go grey.

8 FITTED BLACK AND WHITE T-SHIRTS

A plain, fitted good quality **T-SHIRT** is essential in order to create a more relaxed casual feel to this look. Choose the neckline according to your body shape. V or slash necklines for apple, strawberry and hourglass shapes, high neck for straight shapes and any neckline for pear shapes.

9 FITTED BLACK LEATHER JACKET

The style of this is up to you, it can be a classic leather blazer, a cropped biker jacket or a long leather coat – whatever you feel most comfortable in.

> *Tip* Bear in mind this is a very classic, elegant look – so opt for a jacket with clean lines and minimal embellishment.

10 LEGGINGS

Many women's bugbear – but worn in the right way **LEGGINGS** can be a useful addition to your wardrobe. Unless you have long, skinny legs I would suggest wearing leggings as a layer underneath knit dresses or A-line skirts. Team with heels for über-sexy style, or pumps for everyday – a great way to dress up or down a look from day to evening. As a general rule, unless you're Kate Moss I'd stick to black, navy, grey or brown leggings. Keeping them as muted as possible slims down the legs.

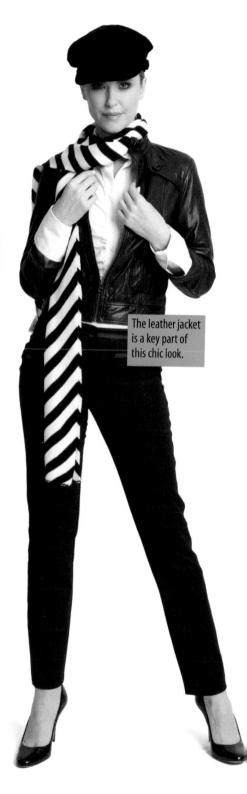

The leather jacket is a key part of this chic look.

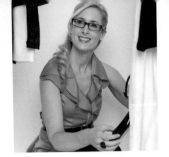
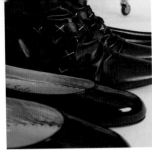
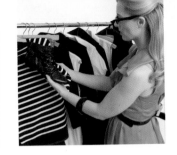

Trimmings

THE ACCESSORIES FOR THIS LOOK ARE AS CLASSIC AS THEY COME. Think Audrey Hepburn meets Jackie O, and indulge your inner superstar.

✦ RED TOTE BAG

Audrey is renowned for her fashionable arm candy, especially her favourite Louis Vuitton TOTE. If you don't want to shell out for the latest IT bag, opt for a high street version instead which is often just as good... and a whole lot more affordable.

✦ BLACK PATENT BALLET PUMPS

Ideal for creating a chic, practical look, these PUMPS can be teamed with just about every element of this look.

✦ BLACK PATENT ROUND COURT SHOES

For a smarter, more sophisticated look sling on a pair of classic, high-heeled COURTS. The round toe perfectly complements and softens this trend.

✦ FLAT POINTED BOOTS

Wear with skinny jeans tucked in, or team with a knit dress or skirt for an elegant but practical look.

✦ BLACK BERET

For that oh-so-French twist, this is a strong Beatnik element.

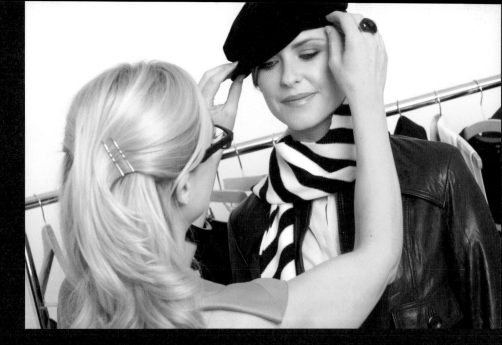

✦ BAKER-BOY CAP
For a casual, street look, swap the beret for a BAKER-BOY CAP instead.

✦ STRIPED NECK SCARF
Ideal if you don't want to go the whole hog and wear a striped jumper but still want to add pattern detailing, without detracting from the overall look.

✦ SLIM BLACK BELT
Worn on the waist or hips, depending on your body shape, a skinny black patent BELT will be a good investment for years to come.

✦ PATTERNED TIGHTS
Another way of introducing a subtle amount of pattern into this look. Best for those with slim legs; black opaque tights are an easier-to-wear alternative.

✦ LARGE SUNGLASSES
Preferably in black – the bigger the better!

✦ LONG GOLD NECKLACE
For a touch of must-have glamour.

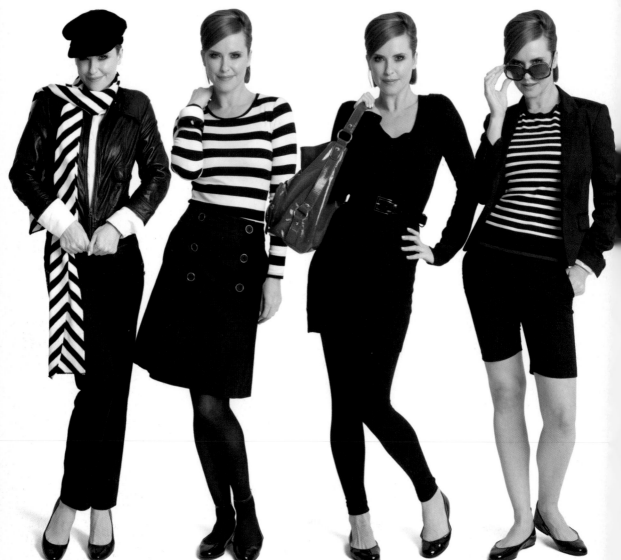

✦ The leather jacket + black trousers + striped scarf

✦ The black and white jumper + A-line skirt + opaque tights

✦ The black knitted dress + skinny black belt + red tote bag

✦ The fitted black blazer + striped jumper + sunglasses

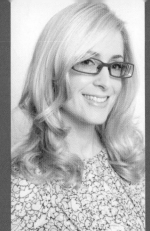

Styling SUGGESTIONS

Now... ACCESSORISE YOUR OUTFIT

	WHITE SHIRT	SLIM BLACK JEANS OR TROUSERS	BLACK KNITTED DRESS	BLACK & WHITE STRIPED JUMPER	BLACK POLO NECK	BLACK A-LINE SKIRT	FITTED BLACK BLAZER	BLACK & WHITE T-SHIRTS	BLACK LEATHER JACKET	LEGGINGS	Now... ACCESSORISE YOUR OUTFIT
1	✓	✓									SKINNY BLACK BELT, BLACK COURT SHOES, GOLD NECKLACE
2			✓							✓	BALLET PUMPS
3		✓		✓					✓		BALLET PUMPS, RED TOTE BAG, STRIPED SCARF, BERET
4					✓	✓	✓				BLACK HEELS, PATTERNED TIGHTS, RED TOTE BAG
5		✓					✓	✓			FLAT BOOTS, STRIPED SCARF, RED TOTE BAG
6	✓	✓									BLACK BERET, BLACK & WHITE STRIPED SCARF, FLAT POINTED BOOTS, RED TOTE BAG
7						✓		✓	✓		BLACK OPAQUE TIGHTS, HEELS, GOLD NECKLACE
8		✓			✓		✓				SKINNY BLACK BELT WITH A BIG SILVER OR GOLD BUCKLE
9			✓						✓		OPAQUE TIGHTS, HEELS
10	✓					✓					PATTERNED TIGHTS, HEELS, LONG GOLD NECKLACE

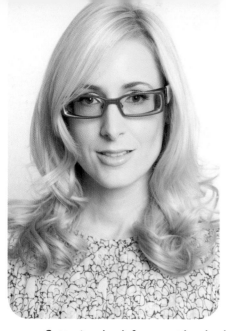

Wear it
YOUR WAY

ALTHOUGH THIS LOOK IS PERHAPS BEST SUITED TO PETITE WOMEN, the monochrome shades make it an extremely flattering look for most body shapes. Head-to-toe black can be severe, but splashes of white or simple accessories will make it much more wearable:

Pear Shapes
(carry weight on their hips and bum):

- ✦ Avoid skinny jeans as they will only emphasise your hips and bottom. Bootcut styles balance out hips and ankles and create the illusion of longer, leaner legs.
- ✦ Flared sleeves will also help to balance out bottom-heavy figures.

Apple Shapes
(carry weight on their tummy and chest):

- ✦ Knitted dresses should be flared from under the bust so that fabric does not cling. If the dress is plain, wear with patterned tights or leggings to show off your legs.
- ✦ Skinny jeans flatter apple shapes as they're great for slim pins. With a tucked-in shirt, swap your slim belt for a wide black belt that sits right over the tummy and hips.

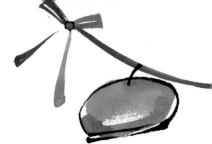

Hourglass
(curvaceous all over with a small waist):

- Polo neck and crew neck tops do not suit women with big busts – period! Always wear either a low scoop or V-neck fitted black jumper to create a flattering shape and highlight your slim waist. In winter, fill in the empty space with a long skinny scarf.
- Where possible wear a skinny belt to draw attention towards your slim waistline.

Boy/Straight (tall and lacking in curves):

- Tall, slim figures are perfect for the polo neck and skinny jeans combo; however, always wear with a skinny black belt to break up the torso and stop it from looking too long and straight.
- You can pull off true Audrey style by wearing black leggings with a long white shirt and ballet pumps. Make sure the shirt is slightly fitted at the waist and then flares out into a stylish shape.
- Make sure your blazer is fitted with slim lapels and collar. Wide styles will only swamp you. A slight nip in at the waist will create the illusion of more shape.

Strawberry Shapes
(broad shoulders and a wide back):

- Avoid polo necks at all costs and stick with fitted V-neck black jumpers or black wrap tops to draw the eye down the body.
- A-line skirts add volume and balance out proportions.
- Patterned tights are fantastic for showing off slim pins.

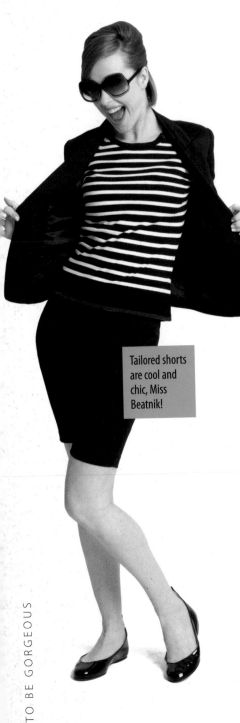

Tailored shorts are cool and chic, Miss Beatnik!

Seasoning

THIS LOOK IS LESS OBVIOUSLY INFLUENCED BY THE SEASONS THAN THE OTHER LOOKS FEATURED IN THIS BOOK. That said, there are a few optional extras that can be introduced to your wardrobe during the year to really make you a Beatnik belle:

Spring/Summer

1. BLACK CAPRI PANTS
2. BLACK COTTON CAPE-STYLE JACKET
3. BLACK AND WHITE STRIPED, FITTED T-SHIRT
4. SLEEVELESS WHITE SHIRT
5. PLAIN WHITE SHIFT DRESS
6. HIGH-WAISTED BLACK SHORTS

Autumn/Winter

1. BLACK MILITARY-STYLE WINTER COAT
2. LONG KNITTED STRIPED WOOL SCARF
3. VELVET BAKER-BOY CAP
4. BLACK WAISTCOAT
5. BLACK WOOL DRESS
6. WIDE, BLACK PATENT BELT
7. TAILORED BLACK WINTER SHORTS
8. BLACK OPAQUE TIGHTS

RECIPE FOR *Success*

THE BEATNIK LOOK ITSELF IS BASED ON A MINIMAL, CLASSIC WARDROBE that can be dressed up and down to suit any body shape, lifestyle and occasion. Just channel Ms. Hepburn and you'll find the world's your movie set.

1. Work

A white shirt worn tucked into a black A-line skirt, patterned tights and black patent heels will look smart and stylish. For a more casual job, wear a black polo neck with either black jeans or trousers and add black patent ballet pumps.

2. Drinks After Work

Finding an outfit that takes you through from a.m. to p.m. need not be a challenge. A black knitted dress with patterned tights and black patent heels works for either the day-shift or drinks with friends; or try a white shirt tucked into black trousers with a long gold necklace.

3. Family Get-Together

Don't want to go overboard but still want to make an effort for the family? A knitted dress with black opaque tights and patent ballet pumps or flat, pointed knee-high boots is the perfect option.

4. Party

To make heads turn wear black slim-leg trousers with sky-high black heels and a sharp tailored white shirt with a long gold necklace and slim belt, or simply pair a LBD with cobweb tights for that certain *je ne sais quoi*.

FINISHING TOUCHES
Make-Up Masterclass

WHEN IT COMES TO 1950S BEATNIK-INSPIRED BEAUTY, IT'S ALL ABOUT SULTRY DOE EYES . . . Audrey Hepburn may have been naturally blessed with her striking eyes, to-die-for skin and famous brows, but you can capture her coquettish essence with my simple make-up tips:

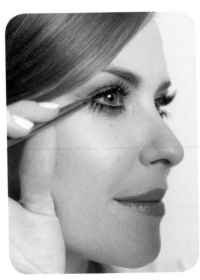

1. Doe Eyes

Now's the time to reach for your mascara, kohl pencil and false lashes! In 1957, Helena Rubinstein introduced the world's first tube and wand applicator mascara, and Beatnik beauties haven't looked back since.

✦ Apply subtle shading to the eye socket using a light taupe brown colour from the lash line to the crease of the socket.
✦ Sweep a highlighter to the brow bone.
✦ Delicately pull your eye taut, and then draw across with black liquid liner in one continuous line from the inner to the outer corner of the eye.

- ✦ Run a black kohl pencil over the lash line to eliminate any gaps.
- ✦ Coat your lashes with three layers of black thickening mascara, starting at the base and zigzagging the colour up to the tip.
- ✦ For really ooh-la-la lashes, fake it! For a more natural look buy individual lashes and add three to the outer corner of the eye.
- ✦ Finish with a pale pout – choosing a lipstick shade roughly the colour of your lips.

Drop Dead Hair

IN THE 1950S SHORT HAIR BECAME CUTTING EDGE. Even today, fashionistas like Erin O' Connor and Agyness Deyn prove that short hair is easy, breezy and fun. Here are some tips on how to achieve three looks from one crop.

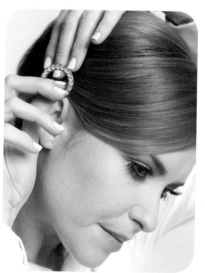

- ✦ *Casual Crop:* Create a tousled, sexy look by working wax or sculpting serum through the layers.
- ✦ *Sophisticated Crop:* Fashion a bold and sleek look by styling damp hair into place. Before it dries, set with strong-hold hairspray and let the style dry naturally.
- ✦ *Glamorous Crop:* Sweep your fringe to the side and secure with a glitzy hair pin. Alternate the side to which you wear your fringe.

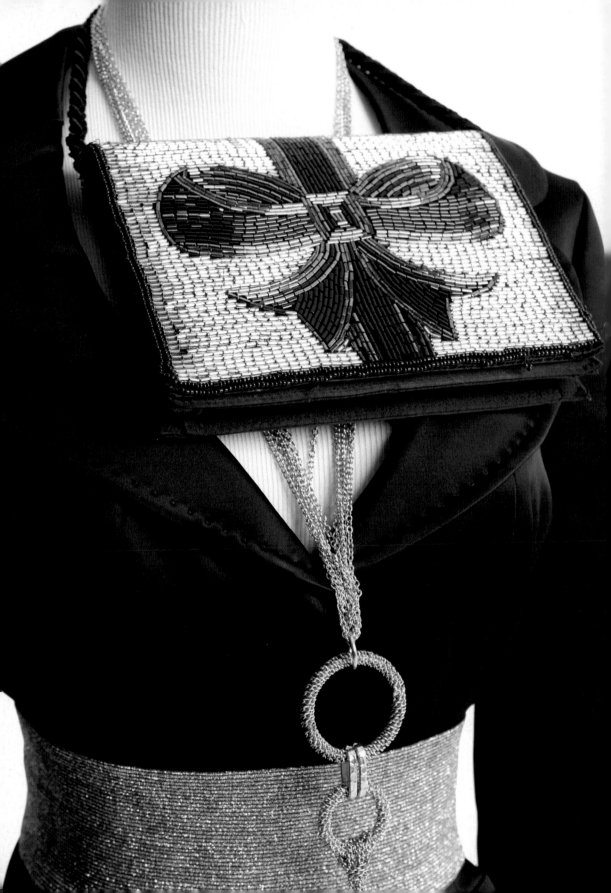

Disco

FUN, FRESH AND DEFINITELY FUNKY, DISCO DIVAS
KNOW HOW TO LIVE IT UP 70S STYLE.

LET'S *Dance*

REMEMBER THE CULT MOVIE *SATURDAY NIGHT FEVER*? For John Travolta and co., **DISCO** was all about youth, optimism and the desire to dance the night away. What better way to forget the pent-up energy of the working week than by dressing up for a night on the town in kick-ass clothing inspired by space and the future?

This look is all about excess: huge platform shoes, glittery make-up (for men too!) and bags of confidence. In terms of clothes, reflective stretch fabrics such as gold lamé, shiny Lycra, Spandex and Lurex are all perfect for posing in under the heady atmosphere of strobe lighting and spinning mirror balls.

Inspiration
FROM THE A-LIST

KNOWN WORLDWIDE FOR HER FIGURE-HUGGING, SHIMMERING STAGE OUTFITS, BEYONCÉ KNOWLES epitomises modern day **DISCO** fashion that takes elements of dancewear and combines it with sexy club styles to achieve eye-popping modern glamour.

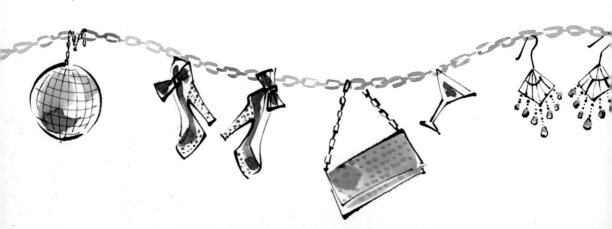

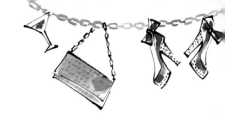

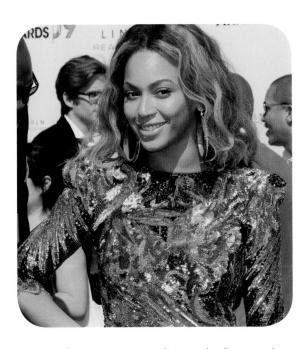

In true show-stopping diva style, Beyoncé has a team of no fewer than twelve people working on her look. However, with the launch of her own fashion label, she's also all about giving ordinary women confidence to shake their thing on the dance floor.

Beyoncé has helped to reshape the **DISCO** look for the new millennium, with more skin on show than ever before, bling accessories and an abundance of colour. What's more, this Disco Diva manages to stay sexy without going over the top by selecting styles that suit her fabulous frame, while her metallic eyes, glossy lips and bronzed cheeks mean her face always radiates.

'I ALWAYS TALK ABOUT FASHION IN MY LYRICS. THE CLOTHES AREN'T MADE JUST FOR THE STAGE, THEY'RE MADE FOR WOMEN WHO WANT TO FEEL LIKE SUPERSTARS AND HAVE EYES ON THEM WHEN THEY WALK INTO A ROOM.'
Beyoncé

Key INGREDIENTS

DON'T BE SCARED! THIS LOOK IS ALL ABOUT GLAMOUR AND GLITZ, which means that adding just a few Disco-inspired pieces to your existing wardrobe will immediately add a show-stopping element to your style. Try these staples for size.

1 METALLIC DRESS

Silver, gold, bronze – metallic fabrics are a big element of this trend. A **METALLIC SHIFT DRESS** will give you the glam factor while still being versatile enough to wear out on a Saturday night, or to a cocktail party. Stretchy knits and satins are more likely to cling, so a heavier weighted fabric with chainmail or sequins can be more forgiving.

> *Tip*
>
> *Keep the balance right – if you're wearing a short dress don't choose one with a low-cut top. Looking sexy is all about leaving something to the imagination!*

2 JEWEL-EMBELLISHED DRESS/TUNIC

This is a great alternative to the metallic dress. It's got the bling factor without the sting. For a classy look, opt for a dress with embellishment just along the neckline. Although black is striking, purple, emerald green and ruby red will have a stronger impact. Keep accessories to a minimum, and let the detail on the dress do the talking. Best teamed with sexy black satin/patent stilettos and matching clutch.

3 SATIN COWL-NECK TOP

This look is all about fabrics with a sheen. A **SATIN TOP** will perfectly complement this look, and the cowl neckline will flatter most body shapes. Team with black trousers/pencil skirt for an evening out or jeans for drinks with friends.

> *Tip* *SATIN can be a tricky fabric, so make sure to wear supportive underwear to give you a smoother silhouette, and talcum powder your armpits to avoid sweat patches.*

4 BOOB TUBE

Wear under a jacket for a more elegant option or layer it under a chiffon blouse so the detail on the top shows through without flashing too much flesh. For younger girls with fabulous figures, team with high-waisted trousers or jeans and get ready to set the night on fire! Avoid if you're full-chested as the **BOOB TUBE** will flatten and square your proportions.

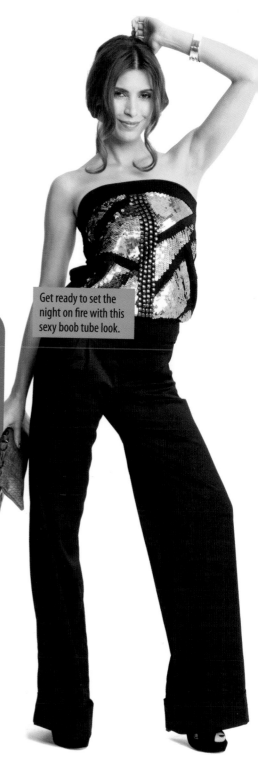

Get ready to set the night on fire with this sexy boob tube look.

5 ONE-SHOULDERED TOP

In true 80s disco style, the **ONE-SHOULDERED TOP** is ideal for any age group – especially if you've got slim arms and shoulders. It's more forgiving than a boob tube, while still super-sexy and feminine. Invest in a good strapless bra that gives you firm support.

6 METALLIC STRAPPY TOP

This is ideal if you don't want to go all out in a metallic dress or boob tube. The **METALLIC STRAPPY TOP** is cool but casual and looks great teamed with jeans and heels for a night out.

> *Tip* *If you've got a pale complexion, try silver metallic tones. For those with olive skin tones, bronzes and golds will work a treat.*

7 LEGGINGS

A throwback from the 80s, **LEGGINGS** are Disco-tastic, and easier to wear than you think. In the past, leggings were teamed with sequined boob tube tops, but for a more modern take, layer under shift dresses/tunics. Black is popular, but for true Disco style, metallic fabrics rule.

8 BLACK SATIN PENCIL SKIRT

A slinky must-have for a night out and the perfect sexy complement to a Disco-style top.

> *Tip* *Opt for a PENCIL SKIRT with a high, wide waistband to draw in your waist and create an hourglass shape.*

9 BLACK SLIM-FIT EVENING TROUSERS

As the majority of tops in this look are bright and bold, it makes sense to pair them with classic basics that won't compete with the look. **BLACK SLIM-FIT TROUSERS** are a great investment for any wardrobe and an essential for this look. If you're conscious of your hips opt for straight or bootleg trousers instead.

10 SATIN BLAZER

Preferably in black for maximum versatility, this **BLAZER** is ideal for toning down sequinned, metallic and boob tube style tops without taking the glamour away from this look. For more formal occasions, team with a pencil skirt and a cowl-neck top.

Tip Definitely worth spending a bit of money on this, as not only will it look expensive it will also go the distance. Cheap satin doesn't wear well.

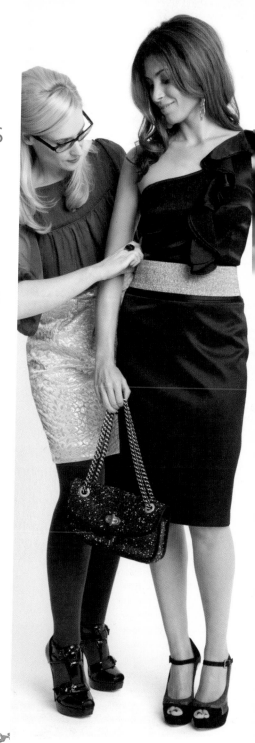

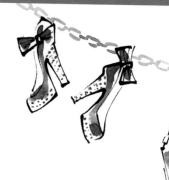

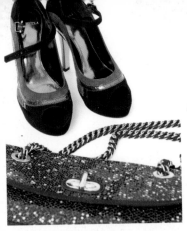

Trimmings

TO SPARKLE ON THE DANCE FLOOR you need to funk up your threads with this bootylicious bling.

✦ CHANDELIER EARRINGS

Long and spangly is great, jewel-encrusted or metallic is a must, but be careful not to overdo the frosting. Ideal with off-the-shoulder tops which elongate the neck and create space for the earrings.

✦ METALLIC WAIST BELT

A METALLIC BELT worn over a black dress or satin top will add a twist of Disco without going over the top.

✦ JEWEL-ENCRUSTED CLUTCH BAG

The perfect accessory for a glam night on the town, but be careful not to go mad with the embellishment. Think 'subtle bling' not 'disco ball'.

✦ STACKS OF GOLD BANGLES

Ideal for the twenty-something. For the rest of us, one or two gold bracelets will be bang on trend, without looking brassy.

✦ DIAMANTÉ NECKLACE

For those of us who can't afford the real thing! Remember, pick one accessory as your focus piece; chandelier earrings plus necklace would be overkill.

✦ LONG, LAYERED GOLD NECKLACES

Keep it to two or three strands at a time – you don't want to be too weighed down to disco!

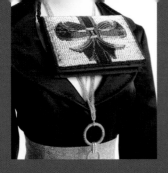 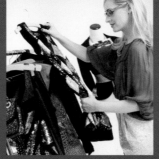 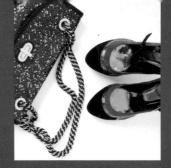

✦ MIRRORED BANGLES

Fantastic if you really want to shine on the dance floor. As a statement piece, these would be best suited to a more muted outfit, such as black slim-fit trousers and satin jacket or a classic LBD.

✦ PLATFORM HEELS

As daunting as they may look, they're often more comfortable than a stiletto heel. PLATFORMS add height and keep the overall look quite young and trendy. Think of them as your personal podium!

✦ METALLIC STRAPPY HIGH SANDALS

The perfect complement to a metallic dress or top. The beauty of metallic accessories is that they complement most shades so you don't need to worry about matching colours and fabrics together.

✦ BLACK, POINTED HIGH HEELS

Ideal for teaming with slim-fit trousers, leggings or dresses with a lot of embellishment as they will add height and elongate the leg without detracting from the look.

✦ SMART BLACK TRENCH COAT

To go over any length dress and keep you warm in the evening when you're queuing to get into a nightclub. Another worthy wardrobe investment, which will become a reliable staple whatever the occasion.

✦ LIP GLOSS

This look is all about a lot of glamour and a touch of GLOSS – don't leave the house without it!

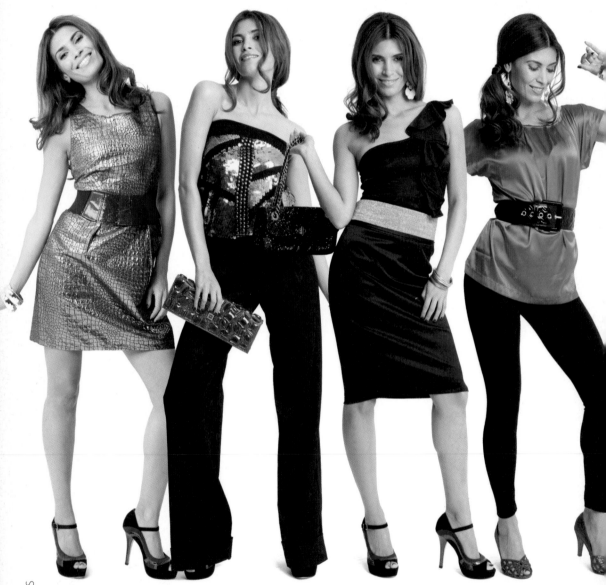

✦ The metalllic dress + platform heel

✦ The boob tube + jewelled clutch

✦ The one - shouldered top + black pencil skirt

✦ The satin tunic + leggings + belt + mirrored bangle

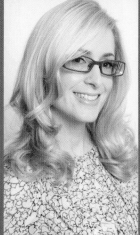

Styling SUGGESTIONS

	METALLIC DRESS	JEWELLED DRESS /TUNIC	SATIN COWL-NECK TOP	BOOB TUBE	ONE-SHOULDERED TOP	METALLIC STRAPPY TOP	LEGGINGS	SLIM BLACK TROUSERS	BLACK SATIN PENCIL SKIRT	SATIN BLAZER	Now... ACCESSORISE YOUR OUTFIT
1				✓				✓		✓	BLACK POINTED HEELS, GOLD BANGLES
2		✓					✓				METALLIC SANDALS, MIRRORED BANGLES
3					✓			✓			CHANDELIER EARRINGS, BLACK POINTED HEELS
4	✓									✓	METALLIC HEELS, LONG GOLD NECKLACES
5			✓					✓		✓	SMALL DIAMANTÉ NECKLACE, METALLIC HEELS
6						✓			✓		BLACK POINTED HEELS, METALLIC BELT, BLACK TRENCH COAT
7			✓					✓			BELT, BLACK HEELS, COUPLE OF BANGLES
8						✓		✓		✓	METALLIC HEELS, CLUTCH BAG CHANDELIER EARRINGS
9		✓						✓			BELT, BLACK HEELS, CLUTCH BAG
10	✓						✓				PLATFORM HEELS, BELT, MIRRORED BANGLE, JEWELLED CLUTCH BAG

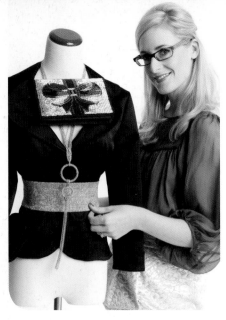

Wear it
YOUR WAY

A STEP UP FROM YOUR 9-5 CLOTHES WILL
MAKE YOU FEEL ULTRA-GLAMOROUS.
Curvaceous, voluptuous or slim, this
eye-catching style can be worn by most body shapes. Feel confident
about yourself, and let your inner **DISCO DIVA** free your figure:

Pear Shapes
(carry weight on their hips and bum):

+ Pencil skirts will only emphasise hips, so choose styles that have a
  wide waistband and flare out over your bottom. Satin reflects light,
  drawing attention to your hips, so opt for a matt stretch fabric instead.
+ Dark denim jeans will look fantastic as long as they are a pure colour
  and do not have faded patches over the thighs. To balance out hips
  don't go for a straight slim-leg; opt for a funky kick-flare instead.

Apple Shapes
(carry weight on their tummy and chest):

+ Swap pencil skirt for a simple black flared skirt with a wide waistband
  or find one with lots of embellished detail around the hemline to
  draw the eye all the way down the body.

- Avoid shoestring tops or boob tubes. Square neckline tops with wide straps will give the impression of bandeau tops in a more flattering shape.

Hourglass
(curvaceous all over with a small waist):

- Use belts to cinch in baggy tops to show off your small waist. If wearing evening trousers or pencil skirt, tuck tops in and accessorise with a metallic belt to accentuate curves.
- Skinny straps on tops can look really strained over big boobs. Instead opt for wider straps to balance out the upper body.

Boy/Straight (tall and lacking in curves):

- Boob tubes look best on tall, straight women with small chests as they help break up the long torso. If you have the figure for it then go to town and choose a colourful, sequined version.
- Watch plunging necklines as they emphasise flat chests. If you dare to bare, go bra-less and wear a backless top for cheeky sex appeal.

Strawberry Shaped
(broad shoulders and a wide back):

- Don't wear boob tubes or tops with shoestring straps as these will look out of proportion on broad shoulders. Try V or cowl necklines with little angel sleeves and wear mirrored bangles for balanced bling.
- Sexy low-cut dresses are Disco-fabulous on you. Draping cowl neck dresses with high waistbands that really flare out to just above the knee will look great too.

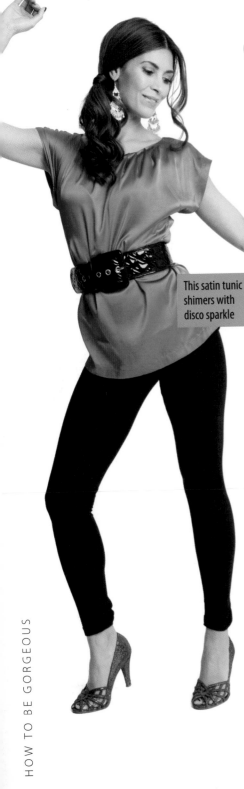

This satin tunic shimers with disco sparkle

Seasoning

PARTY SEASON IS A GREAT TIME FOR WORKING UP A DISCO FEVER, but you don't have to wait for Christmas and New Year to try out this look. With a little imagination, this cheeky style can add a shimmer to your wardrobe all year round:

Spring/Summer

1. PLATFORM SANDALS
2. ANKLE BRACELET
3. SATIN BLOUSE
4. BANDEAU SUNDRESS
5. SWIRLY MAXI DRESS
6. DENIM MINI SKIRT
7. HANDKERCHIEF-STYLE BACKLESS TOP

Autumn/Winter

1. FAKE FUR COAT
2. SHINY HIGH-HEELED BOOTS
3. SATIN TUNIC
4. SLIM-FIT BOOTCUT JEANS
5. ONE-SHOULDERED DRESS
6. BRIGHTLY COLOURED WRAPDRESS

RECIPE FOR *Success*

WHETHER YOUR IDEA OF A GOOD NIGHT OUT INVOLVES BURNING UP THE DANCE FLOOR OR CHILLING WITH FRIENDS, it's always fun to make an effort and feel like a glam goddess. Don't let the term 'Disco' put you off – with some clever styling, this look is more versatile than you think.

1. The Nightclub

The ultimate venue for rocking your disco-glam look! To really shine on the dance floor choose between a metallic or jewel-embellished short dress and team with a pair of black pointed high heels. Layer gold bangles up the arm and don't forget to pack your lip gloss into your jewel-encrusted clutch.

2. The Office Christmas Party

Always a challenge to get the right balance between stand-out and stylish. A metallic dress with black stiletto heels is ideal, but be careful of plunging necklines and deep backs – too much flesh won't get you promoted!

3. The Dinner Party

A toned-down version of Disco is a great look for relaxed dinners with friends. Choose between a bright satin blouse and a simple jewel-encrusted top and pair with black evening trousers for a smart look, or dark jeans, black heels and chandelier earrings for laid-back luxe.

4. The Bar

Opt for dark denim jeans with a simple embellished tunic top or satin blouse and accessorise with black pointed heels and a small pair of earrings. Add a black trench coat to get you snugly and stylishly from A to B.

Make-Up Masterclass

SHE WAS THE LEAD SINGER FOR THE ÜBER-GLAM MUSICAL TRIO DESTINY'S CHILD, she's graced hundreds of magazine covers with her sensational look and she's now a mega star and style icon in her own right – there's no doubt about it, we're *Crazy in Love* with Beyoncé's style. Here's how to recreate her DISCO DIVA look from head to toe.

1. Create the Glow

Beyoncé's make-up usually consists of warm browns to help bring out her luminous skin tone and keep her look natural and glowing. To bring out your own glow, read on.

✦ Apply foundation wherever it's needed – for the most natural look, apply on and around your T-zone, and use an under-eye concealer if necessary.

✦ Next brush a delicate shimmer powder/crème along the top of your cheekbone and a little on the top of your cupid's bow.

✦ For an all-over body glow, apply a shimmering body lotion to décolletage, shoulders and legs.

2. Dancing Eyes

To really stand out on the dance floor, give your delicious diva eyes va va voom by using shimmers, metallic eyeshadows and oodles of voluminous lash!

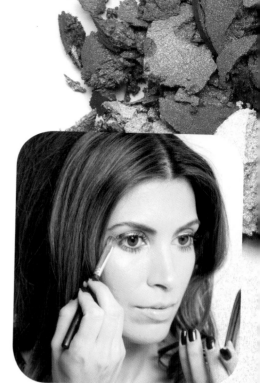

✦ Sweep a shimmering metallic shadow across the eyelid. Then using a pointed eyeliner brush, apply a thin line of the same shadow under the lower lash line.

✦ Apply a dark brown shadow into the crease of the eye starting at the inner corner and working across to the outer corner. Blend well.

✦ Sweep a cream highlighter across brow bones.

✦ Apply brown eyeliner across the upper and lower lash line and gently smudge.

✦ Curl upper lashes using an eyelash curler, then apply dark brown/ black mascara to both upper and lower lashes.

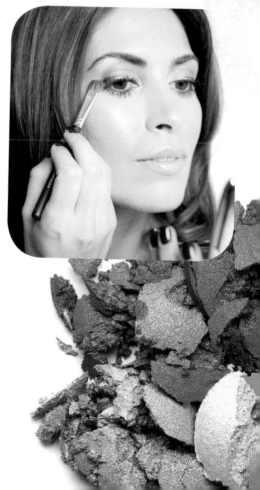

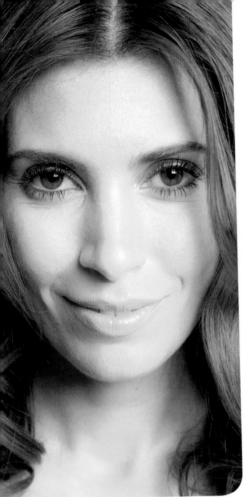

3. Brow Perfect

A DISCO DIVA is always immaculate-looking and few things make a woman appear more groomed than well-plucked eyebrows. I recommend having a professional treatment first to set a 'blueprint', then all you need do is pluck where the hairs grow in. Avoid over-plucking as it can take months for brows to grow back and can be very ageing.

✦ To find where your brows should start, take a pencil and hold it parallel to the side of your nose. Where the brush meets your brow is where your brow should begin.

✦ To find the end of your brow, extend the pencil diagonally from your nostril, following the outside edge of your eye toward the brow. Where the inside edge of the pencil hits is where your brow should end. The best brows have a slight arch. To find yours, hold the brush parallel to the outside edge of the coloured part of your eye. Where the brush meets the brow is where the highest part of your brow should be.

✦ Brush brows into place with a brow gel and fill in any gaps with a brow pencil or taupe shadow.

Drop Dead Hair

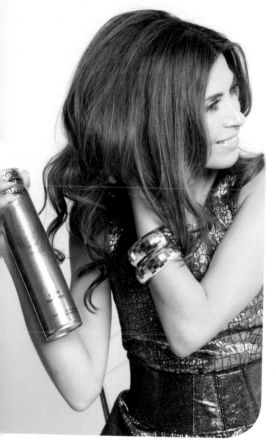

IF YOU REALLY WANT DISCO CHIC, shoulder-length hair or longer is an absolute must! If you don't have long hair, you can always try using clip-in extensions or hair pieces to create a long look of your own. Once you've got the length, you'll want the curls and here's how to get them.

1. Sexy Volume

✦ Begin by shampooing and conditioning hair with a product that is made for your hair type and then towel dry.

✦ Section hair into 1½-inch sections and spray each section with a volumising spray.

✦ Roll each section of hair onto the heated rollers, making sure to roll the hair over the roller as opposed to under to give ultimate volume.

✦ Allow each individual roller to cool. Once the rollers have cooled, carefully remove them and then gently run your fingers through your hair.

✦ To finish this look, mist hair with a holding spray.

chapter 7

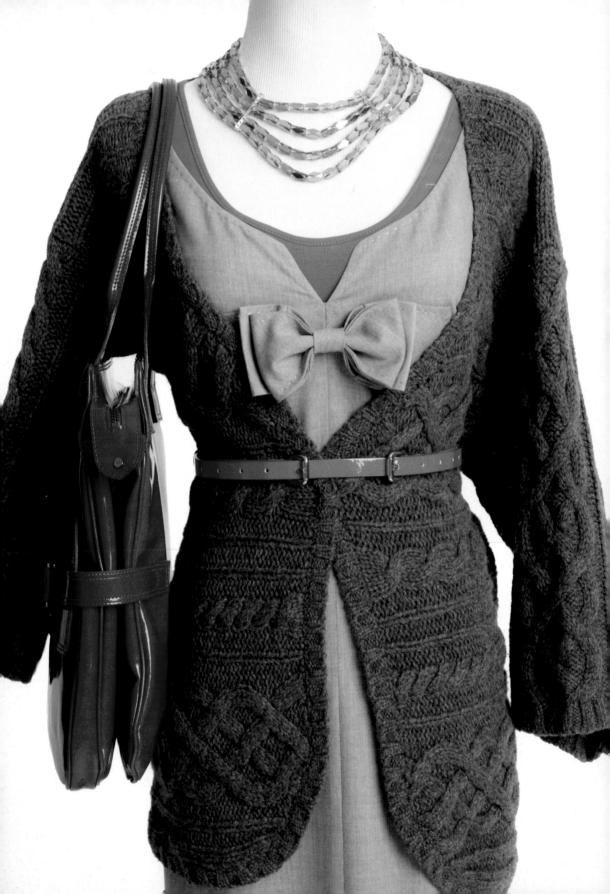

Tailoring

DUST OFF THAT POWER SUIT
AND KILLER HEELS AND SHOW THE WORLD
THAT YOU MEAN BUSINESS!

GIRL *Power*

UNLESS YOU WORK IN THE CORPORATE WORLD, SNAPPY SUITS ARE JUST FOR INTERVIEWS, RIGHT? THINK AGAIN! This 80s-inspired style is all about standing tall in a man's world. Tailoring enables a woman to impart an elegance and sophistication well beyond her years, and disguise indiscretions accumulated over years gone by – which probably explains why it's always been such a powerful force in the history of style.

The 1980s marked the emergence of 'Power Dressing' and the introduction of female tailoring. Young, upwardly mobile professionals (better known as 'Yuppies') were climbing the career ladder and for the first time in history women were battling their way to the top too. Women meant business and the suit was their symbol of the moment that empowered them to achieve their goals.

Sleek & SOPHISTICATED

ALTHOUGH WE'VE NOW LEFT THE MASCULINE SHOULDER PADS AND HELMET-HAIR BEHIND, women still enjoy the look and feeling of tailored clothes, and their ability to make them seem smart, competent, sophisticated and totally in control. Nowadays, heels, trouser suits, pencil skirts and smart shirts are all staples of the modern woman's wardrobe, and regardless of your age or job, the classic tailored jacket still remains an absolute essential for anyone wanting to dress to impress.

Inspiration
FROM THE A-LIST

PRINCESS DIANA CHANGED FASHION with her trend-setting interpretation of modern **TAILORING.** Tall and willowy, she was a designer's dream; a walking advert for any creation. Once married to Prince Charles and with a team of advisors from Vogue magazine, Diana's day look was transformed from frilly blouses and floral skirts, to smartly cut suits with skirts that daringly showed off her fabulous legs, as well as crisp shirts, tailored jackets and casual blue jeans – the epitome of the devoted wife/mother and modern-day working woman.

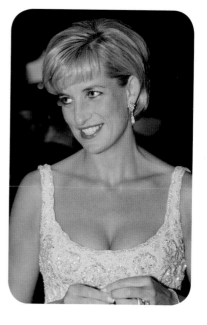

Women felt elevated by Diana's look; she was young, inspiring and what's more her dress sense suited the 30s-50s age group who had been feeling left out by many of the recent fashion trends. Young or old, working girl or stay-at-home mum, Diana's pared-down tailored style gave women inspiration for a smart, together look that exuded the message: Don't underestimate me.

'SHE INNATELY UNDERSTOOD THE POWER OF THE LANGUAGE OF CLOTHES.'

Jasper Conran

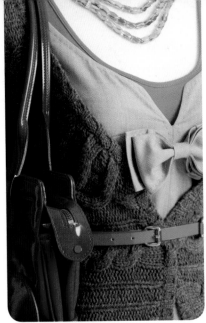

Gorgeous...
NINE TO FIVERS

FLIRTATION, BACK-STABBING, CAMARADERIE AND COMPETITIVENESS . . . and all before the morning meeting! No wonder Hollywood keeps going back to the world of work for their most charming characters and irresistible villains. Here's my list of the ten most inspirational working women:

1. Doralee Rhodes IN NINE TO FIVE

Not only did she write the incredible title song, but perky DOLLY PARTON stars as the ditzy secretary who helps cut her sexist boss down to size in soft pretty knitted dresses that flatter her infamous feminine assets.

2. Betty Draper IN MAD MEN

JANUARY JONES may play a housewife and mother of two, but with her immaculate 60s outfits she provides inspiration for home office bound women everywhere.

3. Tess McGill IN WORKING GIRL

MELANIE GRIFFITH transforms herself from a mild-mannered secretary to a sharply tailored executive thanks to her boss's fabulous designer wardrobe.

4. *M* IN JAMES BOND

The most formidable Bond woman to date, JUDI DENCH keeps James in check, and looks smooth and completely in control in her chic, dark tailored suits.

5. *Isabel Lahiri* IN *OCEANS TWELVE*

In crisp coats and trouser suits, CATHERINE ZETA-JONES manages to stay professional while working alongside Brad Pitt and George Clooney.

6. *Miranda Priestly* IN *THE DEVIL WEARS PRADA*

MERYL STREEP is on supremely icy form as the perfectly coutured editor of a bitchy fashion magazine.

7. *Amanda Tanen* IN *UGLY BETTY*

In the world of *Mode*, image is everything, and BECKI NEWTON's well-groomed receptionist knows it.

8. *Miranda Hobbs* IN *SEX AND THE CITY*

CYNTHIA NIXON's sharp masculine suits mixed with feminine detailing are perfect for the modern board room.

9. *Lois Lane* IN *SUPERMAN*

Running around town in a tight pencil skirt and sky-high heels, TERI HATCHER manages to get the story and the action hero.

10. *Michelle Obama*

THE FIRST LADY of modern 9-5 style, teaching us all the new approach to dressing a.m to p.m and the art of choosing a simple silhouette and statement jewellery.

Key INGREDIENTS

YOU DON'T NEED TO BE A DYNASTY DIVA OR A WALL STREET HOTSHOT TO APPRECIATE THE POWER OF THE TAILORED LOOK. The beauty of tailoring is its simplicity and structure. A well-cut suit needs little embellishment to stand out, and a fitted jacket or pair of tailored trousers will discretely disguise imperfections and remain timelessly stylish. Whatever your 9-5 style, here's how to ensure you've got fail-safe sophistication lined up when you need it.

1 THE WHITE SHIRT

The foundation of any tailored look, preferably fitted with a strong collar. A great way to soften the structure of this look is to invest in a shirt with feminine touches: ruffle details, double cuffs, mandarin necklines, pleating or voluminous sleeves.

2 THE COLOURED TAILORED SHIRT

Great for adding variety and a splash of colour to what is in essence quite a stark, masculine look. Opt for strong colours like hot pink, red, purple and turquoise that will make you stand out.

Tip *Don't be scared to wear a BOLD COLOUR that sets you apart from the masses. If you're not sure whether a colour suits you or not, hold it up to your face. If it lights up your skin - winner!*

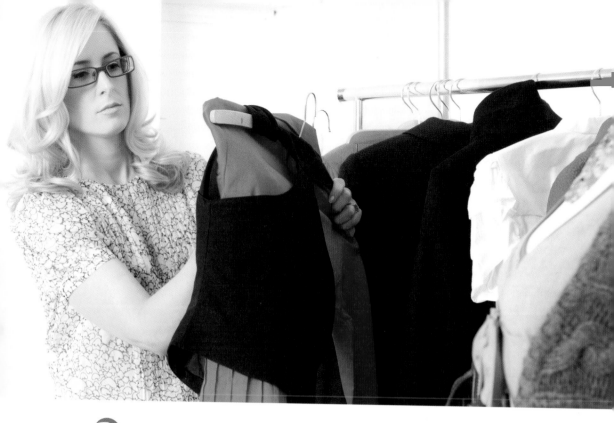

3 SKIRT SUIT

A **SKIRT SUIT** is ideal for the modern woman who wants to balance her ambition against her femininity. Choose the shape of your skirt depending on your body shape. The overall look should be very sharp and sophisticated while still looking feminine and sexy.

4 TAILORED TROUSERS

An essential piece for your tailored look, choose between slim and wide-leg, depending on your body shape and preference. Try to avoid a wardrobe of black trousers – it might make getting dressed easy in the morning but you'll look nondescript. For added variety, include other colours such as navy, brown, grey, white and cream into the mix. It's really worth investing in a couple of good quality, great fitting trousers – not only will they last, but they will offset anything you wear.

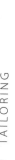

TAILORING

143

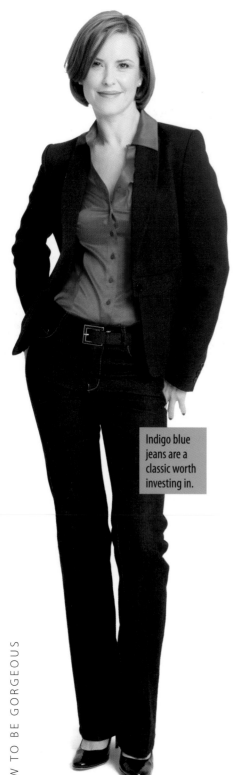

Indigo blue jeans are a classic worth investing in.

5 SMART INDIGO BLUE JEANS

Tailoring is all about classic staples that will go the distance. When it comes to a smart pair of timeless trousers it has to be a pair of dark blue, straight-leg **JEANS**. Smart enough to wear to work with a tailored jacket and heels, casual enough to wear with boots and slouchy cardigan; flattering for any size or shape. Definitely worth spending the money on a good pair of jeans, as pound per wear they will earn their keep. Always wash indigo jeans inside-out to preserve colour and never tumble-dry as this destroys the natural stretch in the fabric.

6 FITTED BLAZER

Look the business in this tailored, casual jacket which you can throw on with jeans over a knit or shirt – one of Princess Di's favourite looks. Avoid anything that looks too corporate and opt for black, navy, white or striped fabric to help differentiate your working wardrobe from your casual one.

7 FITTED SCOOP-NECK STRETCH TOP

Teaming jersey knit tops with softer necklines like a **SCOOP NECK** is an ideal way to feminise a tailored look. It's also an ideal alternative to a fitted shirt, and for travelling as it requires less maintenance to look good.

8 FINE KNITTED JUMPER

Long-sleeved, short-sleeved or sleeveless – quality is key, whichever you choose. These are ideal for layering over fitted shirts for a relaxed, but still professional look.

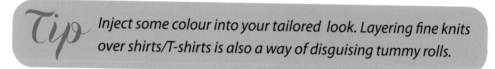

Tip *Inject some colour into your tailored look. Layering fine knits over shirts/T-shirts is also a way of disguising tummy rolls.*

9 WAISTCOAT

A great alternative to the knitted jumper for more formal occasions. You get to create a more fashionable look and you don't have to wear a formal jacket. Waistcoats are brilliant for emphasising waistlines; team with high-waisted wide-leg trousers to conceal tummy bulges. For tall slim frames, layer over voluminous tops to create curves.

10 WRAP DRESS

A **WRAP DRESS** is a must-have as it suits all figures and can be brought in lightweight fabrics in summer and heavier ones in winter. For a more tailored look, opt for a bold plain colour as opposed to one with loud patterns all over. Accessorise with a belt to give it a more modern twist – wrap dresses can look frumpy if not accessorised in the right way.

Trimmings

DON'T GET HOOKED INTO WEARING a black suit and white shirt every day with the same necklace or earrings day in, day out! A few statement accessories will immediately set you apart from the rat race.

✦ SLIM HIPSTER BELT

Black, red or even a wild pink trouser-belt will immediately create a focal point and add an element of style to your look. Ideal for if you want to draw attention away from your waist.

✦ SKINNY WAIST BELT

Layer over high-waisted skirts or jumpers and shirts to define the waist. A SLIM-LINE BELT looks more professional than the wider variety and will immediately break up monotonous colour and create curves.

✦ BLACK OR DARK TAN HIGH-HEELED BOOTS

Boots are infinitely more comfortable than heels, so you can wear a higher heel while still being able to walk. Either wear under trousers, or for a more fashionable look, invest in pair of ankle boots and team with skirts or dresses.

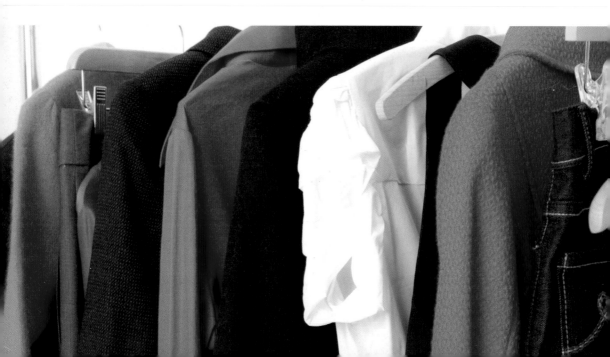

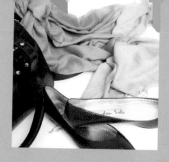
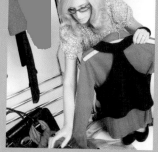
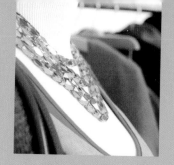

✦ BLACK STILETTO HEELS

Pointed heels help to elongate the leg and give a smart understated look. The round-toe court shoe is a more contemporary look that works with trousers – especially the wide-leg type. Stiletto heels are important because they signify classic elegance that suits any style of tailoring.

✦ CHUNKY SILVER NECKLACE

Perfect for layering over plain jumpers or shirts, particularly polo/cowl neck tops where you can really make the NECKLACE into a feature.

✦ SMALL STUD EARRINGS

Don't feel you have to limit yourself to plain gold studs or pearls. Why not be more adventurous and go for something bolder and more colourful?

✦ LARGE COCKTAIL RING

Another way of injecting a bit of fun into your tailored look, and the perfect accessory to dress up your work suit for evening.

✦ LEATHER STRUCTURED SHOULDER BAG

Perfect for carrying paper files in without the need for a briefcase; also a practical handbag for shopping or playing with the kids at the weekend when you need to keep your hands free.

✦ PASHMINA

The classic Princess Diana accessory; ideal for draping over jackets or dresses for in-between days when you don't want to wear a coat or outdoor jacket.

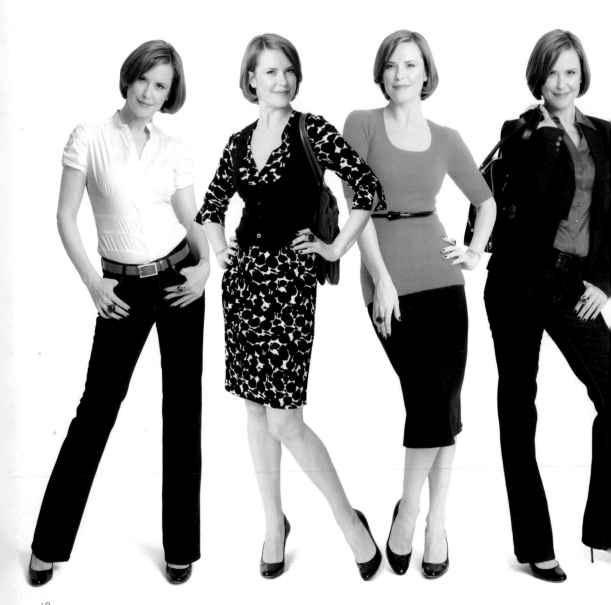

✦ The dark indigo jeans + skinny waist belt + white shirt

✦ The wrap dress + waistcoat + black pointed heel

✦ The fine knitted jumper + skirt suit + black pointed heel

✦ The dark indigo jeans + fitted blazer + slim black belt

Styling SUGGESTIONS

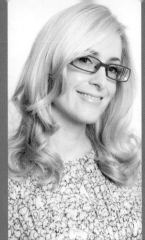

	White Shirt	Coloured Shirt	Skirt Suit	Tailored Trousers	Smart Dark Jeans	Fitted Blazer	Fine Knitted Jumper	Waistcoat	Wrap Dress	*Now...* ACCESSORISE YOUR OUTFIT
1		✓		✓				✓		BLACK POINTED HEELS, CHUNKY SILVER NECKLACE, COCKTAIL RING
2	✓				✓	✓				SLIM BLACK BELT, CHUNKY SILVER NECKLACE, BLACK POINTED HEELS
3	✓		✓							SHOULDER BAG, BLACK POINTED HEELS, SMALL STUD EARRINGS, SLIM WAIST BELT
4	✓			✓			✓			SLIM BELT IN COMPLEMENTARY COLOUR TO KNIT, SMALL STUD EARRINGS, SLIM WAIST BELT
5	✓				✓		✓			SLIM BLACK BELT, POINTED HEELS, CHUNKY SILVER NECKLACE, PASHMINA
6		✓			✓					SLIM BELT, CHUNKY SILVER NECKLACE, COCKTAIL RING, POINTED HEELS
7				✓		✓	✓			BRIGHT PASHMINA, POINTED BOOTS
8		✓			✓			✓		CHUNKY SILVER NECKLACE, SMALL STUD EARRINGS, POINTED HEELS
9						✓			✓	SLIM OR WIDE BLACK BELT, CHUNKY SILVER NECKLACE, POINTED HEELS
10			✓				✓			CHUNKY SILVER NECKLACE, SLIM BLACK BELT, POINTED HEELS

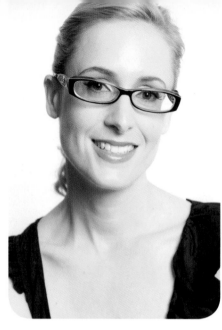

Wear it
YOUR WAY

TO ACHIEVE THE DIANA LOOK, YOU DON'T HAVE TO BE TALL AND SLIM; it's all about proportions and thinking wisely about jacket shapes in particular. The beauty of tailoring is that well-structured clothes will disguise countless imperfections.

Pear Shapes
(carry weight on their hips and bum):

✦ Wide-leg trousers are great for balancing out hips. Make sure they are flat-fronted and have a wide waistband. If they have pockets, get them stitched up to avoid adding any extra width.

✦ Slim belts only emphasise hips so go for a slightly wider style, with a buckle that is not chunky. Wear over your jacket to show off your shape.

✦ For a perfect suit, go for a fishtail skirt that is fitted at the top and then flares out from the knee. The jacket should have wide lapels, be nipped in at the waist and flared over hips to boost shape and definition.

Apple Shapes
(carry weight on their tummy and chest):

✦ Use chunky necklaces to attract attention away from problem areas.

✦ For your ideal suit, ditch the straight pencil skirt in favour of a flared

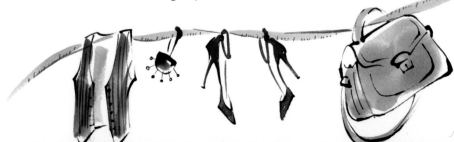

circular style or a more classic A-line cut with a flattering, wide waistband. Keep the jacket cropped with a slight fit and flare and go for two buttons.

Hourglass
(curvaceous all over with a small waist):

✦ Choose cotton shirts that have a small amount of stretch to help mould around bust and waist. Look for styles that are ruched around the buttons as this will help minimise big busts and hide a few extra pounds if needed.

✦ Work your curves in sexy pencil or fishtail skirts and a jacket that is cropped and very fitted at the waist. Help balance the bust by going for wider lapels and a maximum of two buttons to ensure the jacket does not sit too high up on the chest.

Boy/Straight *(tall and lacking in curves):*

✦ Take maximum advantage of your tall, slim figure and show off those pins in a pencil skirt teamed with a narrow-cut jacket that has a very gentle fit and flare.

✦ Wrap dresses should belt high up on the waist to break up torso and even out proportions.

Strawberry Shaped
(broad shoulders and a wide back):

✦ Don't be tempted to do shirt buttons up too high; always leave at least a couple undone – three if it doesn't look too risqué.

✦ Wide-leg trousers will help to balance out your proportions.

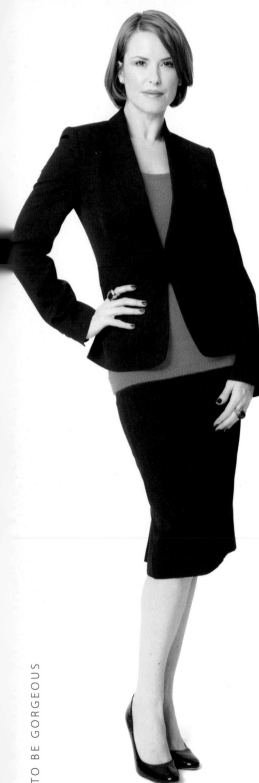

Seasoning

TAILORING IMMEDIATELY LENDS ITSELF TO AUTUMN/WINTER FASHIONS; however, incorporating some structure into your summer wardrobe can give a smart edge to the soft, floaty feminine styles that women so often struggle with. Here are some key pieces to help you dress to impress, whatever the season:

Spring/Summer

1 CITY SHORTS
2 LIGHT COTTON BLAZER
3 SLEEVELESS TAILORED SHIRTS
4 FITTED SHIFT DRESS
5 TAN POINTED HEELS
6 LINEN/COTTON-MIX WIDE-LEG TROUSERS
7 CANVAS STRUCTURED BAG

Autumn/Winter

1 TAILORED, BELTED BLACK WINTER COAT
2 OPAQUE TIGHTS
3 WOOL FLANNEL TROUSERS
4 CHUNKY BELTED WRAP CARDIGAN
5 WIDE BELT
6 HEAVY WOOL BLAZER

RECIPE FOR *Success*

THIS IS A STYLE BEST KEPT FOR DAYWEAR; it's a style perfect for those looking for an easy-to-manage smart image with little fuss and a lot of flair. Here's how to adapt your tailored wardrobe to suit your lifestyle.

1. The Formal Office

Let your personal style shine through in a subtle way by going for a skirt or trouser suit that flatters your body shape and team with a tucked-in, well-tailored shirt and some killer black heels. No one's going to walk all over you in that ensemble!

2. The Casual Office

Go for a fitted blazer in a different fabric but complementary colour to your trousers so that your look is smart, chic and unique.

3. The School Run

Just because you're not at work doesn't mean that you can't dress with a little smart sophistication. Wear jeans with tailored double-cuff shirt tucked in, layer fitted fine-knit V-neck jumper over the top and add pointed boots. Very yummy mummy!

4. Lunch

If you're going to a nice restaurant and you want to make a little effort, the wrap dress is the perfect solution. Make sure it's belted to give definition and shape and wear with black or tan heels and small stud earrings.

FINISHING TOUCHES

Make-Up Masterclass

TO PULL OFF THIS LOOK, it's essential that your make-up reflects the sophistication of your clothes in a chic, groomed and timeless way. Here are some tips to help you achieve a classic look that'll get you promoted in no time.

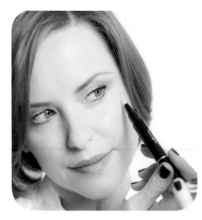

1. Refine Your Bone Structure

Just as you have refined your body shape through the use of clever tailoring, you can do the very same to your facial structure. By contouring the face using bronzer, a clever highlighting pen and a dab of blusher, it is possible to create the illusion of chiselled features and avoid the knife!

✦ Suck in your cheeks to locate your cheekbones, then brush matt bronzing powder under them.

✦ Add bronzer to the bridge of your nose and at the temples.

✦ Brush blush onto the apples of your cheeks. Pull the blush back towards your temples, making the line of brush narrower as you get closer to the hairline.

- Now apply a highlighting pen in a thin stripe down bridge of your nose and blend with your fingertip. Add highlighter around the outer corners of your eyes, top of cheekbones, middle of your chin and temples.

2. Eye-to-Eye

To play up your tailored look, go for simple eye make-up that is individually suited to the shape of your eyes. Use natural hues to keep your overall look classic, groomed and sophisticated.

- If you have ALMOND-SHAPED EYES, create a contrast between the eyelid and the brow bone by using a light shade of eyeshadow from your lashes to your brow, a medium shade on your eyelid, and then a darker shade on the outer third of your eyelid.
- If your eyes are CLOSE TOGETHER you can create an illusion of width by applying eyeliner and dark eyeshadow to the outer third of your lash line and lid.
- Open up DEEP-SET EYES by rimming eyes with smudgy liner, and darkening your eyeshadow slightly above the eyelid crease.
- To make WIDE-SET EYES appear closer together, use a darker shade of eyeshadow in the inner corner of the eyelid and blend this up and out to just underneath the brow bone. Finish with mascara, applying it more heavily on the inner corner of the eye.
- To elongate ROUND EYES, apply eyeliner to both the top and bottom eyelids, extending the liner just beyond the outer corners. With your eyeshadow, focus the light colour on the outer section of the eyebrow bone making sure that it is brushed outwards.

Drop Dead Hair

YOUR SLEEK, TAILORED LOOK
DESERVES A SIMPLE SOPHISTICATED
STYLE THAT EXUDES CONFIDENCE.

Nothing screams 'success' like salon-fresh hair, but here are a few tips on how to look like a high-flyer, however rushed you are.

1. The French Twist

A simple, elegant and timeless up-do that's ideal for long hair, and perfect for the tailored look.

- Use a brush or comb to sweep your hair back from your forehead. Gather hair loosely at the base of your neck, holding hair about three inches from ends.
- Lift your hair so that the ends are pointing up. Twist your hair to the right to create a twist or roll effect at the back of the neck.
- Hold the ends with your left hand and twist the hair tighter until it feels secure.
- Use your right hand to fold the ends of your hair over, down toward

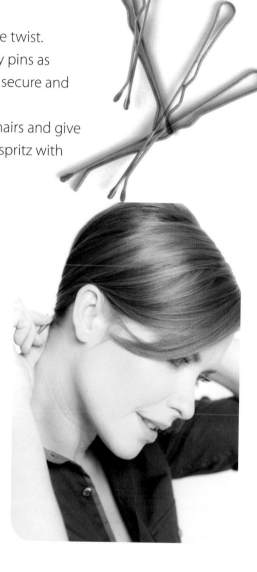

the base of your neck, and under the twist.

- ✦ Pin hair in place. Use as many bobby pins as is necessary to give the twist a nice, secure and tight feel.
- ✦ Use a glossing wax to control stray hairs and give your hair a healthy, shiny look, then spritz with maximum-hold hairspray.

2. The Diana Crop

Very short hair is one of the most neat and chic styles to sport. Princess Diana's hair always exuded femininity and sophistication by keeping a little length at the nape of her neck. One easy method for styling very short hair is to simply slick it back. This look adds easy sophistication with absolutely no hassle.

- ✦ Squeeze a generous amount of hair gel into your palm, and rub your palms together.
- ✦ Starting with the hair closest to your face, slick back through damp hair.
- ✦ Let hair dry naturally.

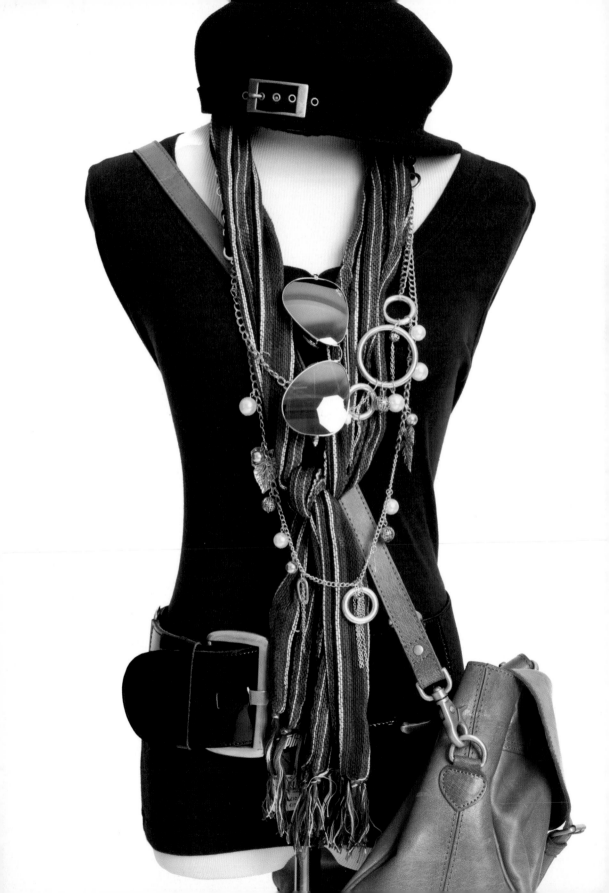

chapter 8

Top Gun

IF YOU FEEL THE NEED TO SPEED YOURSELF INTO
THE FASHION ELITE, WHY NOT JOIN THE RANKS OF
THE MILITARY FASHIONISTAS?

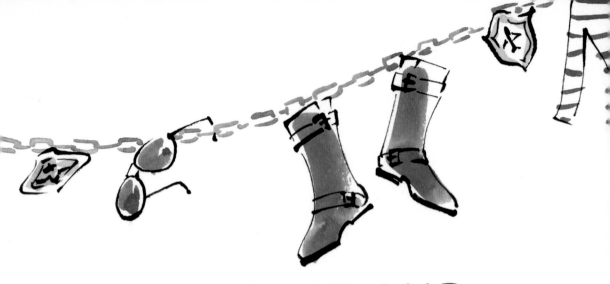

ALL PRESENT AND
Correct

EVER SINCE ELVIS PRESLEY GOT THE G.I. BLUES, CELEBRITIES AND CIVILIANS ALIKE HAVE BEEN TAKING INSPIRATION FROM THAT MOST UTILITARIAN OF DRESS STYLES: military uniform. Wars may come and go, but Top Gun style still claims its place on the catwalk year after year, making it a classic wardrobe staple. What most people don't realise is just how much of an influence military history has on the way we dress. From khakis to bell-bottoms, bomber jackets to aviator sunglasses, regimental tartans to army camouflage, designers have frog-marched uniforms out of the parade ground and onto the catwalk.

With the high street keeping hot on the coat-tails of this style, women of all ages are drawn to the easiness and practicality of the **MILITARY** look. Besides old faithfuls like combats and the utility jacket, the eye-catching embellishment and fine tailoring of servicemen's clothes have redefined classic day glamour for a new generation of shipshape women.

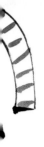

Inspiration
FROM THE A-LIST

DRESSED UP OR DOWN, this look is easy to throw together for a dash round the shops or a sweep down the red carpet. While Gwen Stefani rocks her army fatigues with skimpy vests and plenty of bling, Fearne Cotton prefers to mix her Napoleon-inspired jacket with pretty punk pieces . . . but the one star that really earns fashion wings for her take on soldiers style is **ERIN O'CONNOR**

Famous for her androgynous model look, Erin has always made the most of her figure by wearing masculine-inspired clothes with a slight feminine twist. The trench, skinny trousers, the man's shirt buttoned right up and her trademark flat cap are all wardrobe staples that work well with her sharp, tailored adaptation of the Military trend. To pull off Military chic, take elements of service-men's uniforms and mix them up with both masculine and feminine shapes to create a subtle, glamorous edgy look that need not break the bank.

'I HAVE GROWN UP WITH A SORT OF EMOTIONAL LOYALTY CARD TO THE HIGH STREET. I GET AS MUCH SATISFACTION RUSHING TO TOPSHOP AS I DO RECEIVING THE LATEST FREEBIE FROM PRADA.'

Erin O-Connor

Key INGREDIENTS

WHETHER YOU'RE AWARE OF IT OR NOT, THE CHANCES ARE YOU ALREADY HAVE SOME KEY MILITARY STAPLES IN YOUR CLOSET, and just need some help styling them for a fresh Top Gun twist. The trick is in the detail: epaulettes on shirts and jackets, brass buttons or braiding on coats, double pockets on jackets and trousers, with red, black, navy and khaki being the military colour code. Here are my top ten military essentials.

1 COMBAT TROUSERS

Before you get too excited, let me make myself quite clear that a wardrobe full of **COMBAT TROUSERS** does not qualify as military style! To avoid looking like a lazy dresser be sure to team combats with a fitted top or jacket and wear with heels, Madonna-style, for a more elegant finish. If you have heavy thighs avoid combats with heavy pocket detailing and opt instead for zip pockets.

2 TRENCH COAT

Whether you want a funnel neck, mandarin collar, large buttons or concealed buttons, always choose the style according to your body shape. All styles should be belted and knee-length – you can always tie the belt at the back and wear open to create a long, slim line.

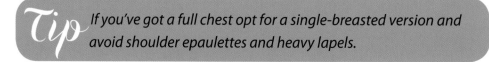

Tip *If you've got a full chest opt for a single-breasted version and avoid shoulder epaulettes and heavy lapels.*

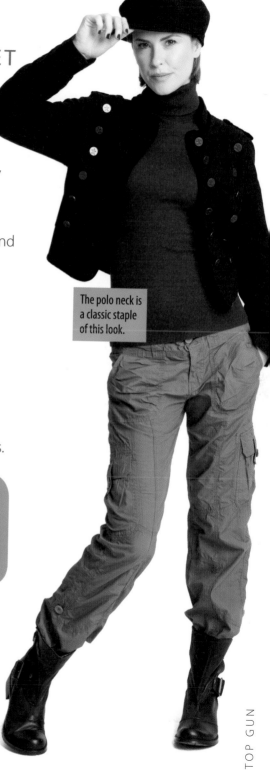

The polo neck is a classic staple of this look.

3 NAPOLEON JACKET

Go long, or opt for a fitted, cropped military-style jacket with a mandarin collar. These jackets have rows of buttons down the front and sometimes hook-and-eye fastenings. They look fantastic teamed with jeans or wide-leg trousers. Best suited to pear or straight shapes who have smaller chests and slim waists.

4 SHIRT WITH EPAULETTES

Look for one in white or khaki tones, with or without a collar and with signature military epaulettes on the shoulders. Fitted usually looks more flattering, but baggy and belted also works.

Tip *Avoid epaulettes if you're broad shouldered; opt instead for combat trousers and a classic fitted shirt for a military twist.*

5 POLO NECK

This original winter warmer is now a classic staple in many women's

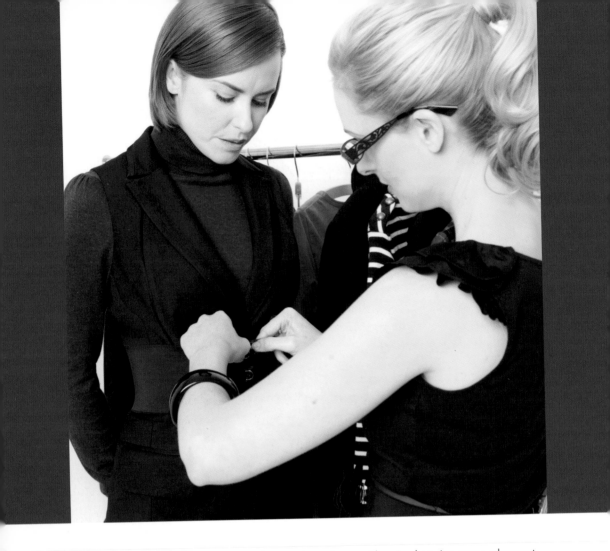

wardrobes. Worn on its own or layered underneath a jacket, its easy, elegant style means it can be dressed up or down, taking you effortlessly from day to dinner. Go for a black or dark khaki tone to really maximise wearability.

6 LONG-LINE WAISTCOATS

Military-style waistcoats are generally hip length and often have a belt around the waist – think safari suit. This is a great piece to carry you between seasons. It can be worn as a top over jeans or a pencil skirt or as a jacket over a long-sleeved top or shirt.

7 TARTAN

Get ready to join the Tartan Army! **TARTAN** is not just for girls in their teens as the variety of brights and muted colours means it works for all age groups. If, however, you want something more subtle, then opt for a bag or a headband that nods towards the look.

> *Tip* *If you find a tartan item that flatters your figure, don't get rid of it as soon as it falls out of fashion. Just store it away until the next time the trend comes round again.*

8 SLIM-LEG TROUSERS

Stand to attention in chocolates, black, even very dark khaki tones, and woollen fabrics too. Ideal for teaming with Napoleon jackets, oversized cardigans and long-line waistcoats.

9 MILITARY COAT

It's definitely worth investing in a military-style **COAT,** either in a belted or A-line shape. Black or red are the classic colours but purple and greens will also make a style statement. The great thing about a military coat is that it makes anything look smart and chic; wear over a dress with heels or over boots tucked into jeans – the perfect alternative to a baggy fleece.

10 BUCKLED BOOTS

Flat and masculine with heavy treads or heeled, pointy and elegant, either way **BOOTS** with buckle detail are the must-have footwear for completing the **TOP GUN** look. Go for knee-length black or chocolate versions and wear with jeans tucked in.

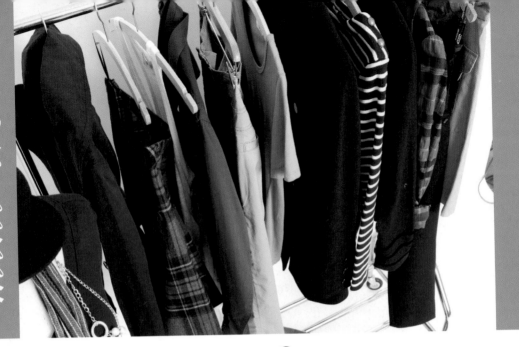

NAUTICAL & SAFARI

SHARP MILITARY TAILORING IS ALL FINE AND DANDY, but don't forget the other elements to the trend: nautical gear and crisp, cool safari style.

1 CLEAR THE DECKS FOR YOUR HOLIDAY WARDROBE – Most of us only get one or two real breaks a year, so make the most of your time in the sun by updating your look. A navy bikini, striped sundress and comfortable deck shoes will have you looking nautical and nice, without going overboard.

2 KEEP COOL – The army have special uniforms for working in warm climates, so why shouldn't you? Avoid looking hot and harassed in the summer months by swapping your heavy, tailored jacket for a light safari suit. Wide-brimmed hat strictly optional!

3 FLY THE COLOURS – From dark blues to soft stones and beiges – what makes the nautical and safari looks so wearable are the gorgeous palettes of colour they use.

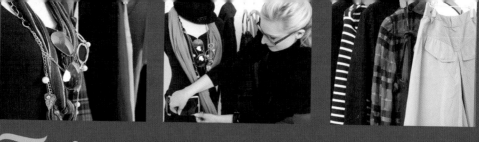

Trimmings

IF YOU REALLY WANT TO PULL OFF THIS LOOK with flying colours here are some optional extras worth considering:

✦ FLAT CAP

As worn by Erin – will complete your look, but make sure to keep it simple and chic. Keep it black, in either felt or wool so it'll hold its shape and last you for many years.

✦ ELASTICATED BUCKLE BELT

The beauty of this BELT is that you can wear it over your military jacket to cinch in the waist or low on your hips over a shirt tucked into trousers.

✦ SATCHEL

Look for a men's utility bag, in beaten dark chocolate or black leather.

✦ SKINNY SCARF

For this look go for a muted khaki tone and wear it knotted around the neck with your shirt and trench coat. Avoid wearing with jackets that have detailing or polo necks as the clean silhouette of this look will be lost.

✦ CHUNKY CHAINS

Choose between gold and silver chunky necklaces and bracelets. The best are those with military influenced charms such as anchors or faux medals.

✦ AVIATOR SUNGLASSES

Make like Tom Cruise in the ultimate military-influenced eyewear.

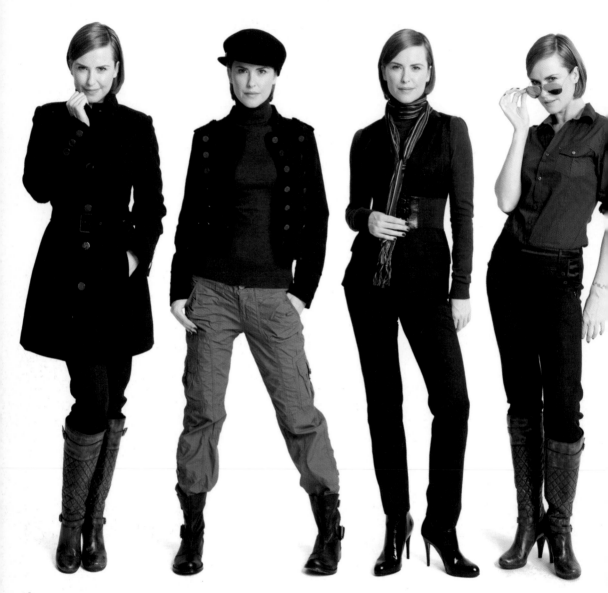

✦ The trench coat + knee-high buckled boots

✦ The combat trousers + buckled boots + polo neck

✦ The long-line waistcoat + slim-leg trousers + polo neck

✦ The slim-leg trousers + military shirt + aviators

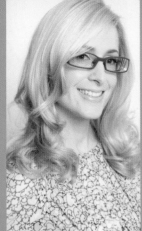

Styling
SUGGESTIONS

Now... ACCESSORISE YOUR OUTFIT

	Combat Trousers	Military Shirt	Napoleon Jacket	Slim-Leg Trousers	Polo Neck	Long-Line Waistcoat	Tartan	Military Coat	Trench Coat	Now... ACCESSORISE YOUR OUTFIT
1	✓		✓		✓					POINTED BOOTS AND BELT
2		✓		✓					✓	BUCKLE BOOTS, BELT AND SKINNY SCARF
3					✓		✓	✓		TARTAN SKIRT, HEELED BUCKLE BOOTS AND SATCHEL
4				✓		✓	✓			TARTAN SHIRT, POINTED BOOTS AND BELT
5				✓	✓				✓	BUCKLED BOOTS, BELT AND FLAT CAP
6		✓		✓	✓					BUCKLED BOOTS AND BELT
7	✓				✓	✓				POINTED BUCKLE BOOTS AND SATCHEL
8	✓				✓			✓		HEELED, POINTED BOOTS AND BELT
9				✓			✓			TARTAN SHIRT, HEELED BUCKLED BOOTS, BELT, SATCHEL
10		✓	✓	✓						HEELED OR FLAT POINTED BOOTS, FLAT CAP

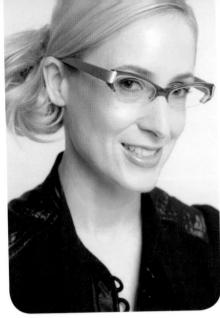

Wear it
YOUR WAY

ALTHOUGH TOP GUN FASHION IS BASED ON MASCULINE SHAPES it does not mean that you need to have a waif-like body or tomboy style to achieve the look. Think of it more as making a strong, confident style statement. Here's how to make Military work for you:

Pear Shapes
(carry weight on their hips and bum):

✦ Really play up your slim upper body with shirts buttoned up high with big epaulettes, button detailing and bold prints like tartan.

✦ Always wear combat trousers with heels and avoid any large zip detailing over hips and thighs. Never go for bold camouflage prints as these will only emphasise width across your bottom.

Apple Shapes
(carry weight on their tummy and chest):

✦ Trench coats and jackets with belts usually sit right on the waist, which focuses in on rounded tummies. Always wear belts tied up at the back to create a long lean shape at the front of the body.

✦ Avoid double-breasted military jackets as these will simply add bulk

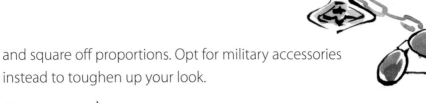

and square off proportions. Opt for military accessories instead to toughen up your look.

Hourglass
(curvaceous all over with a small waist):

✦ Collarless or mandarin collars feature quite heavily in military jackets, but if you leave them open the jacket does not lay well over big busts. To avoid this do the bottom buttons up to create a more flattering shape, or opt for a jacket with wide lapels instead.

✦ Do a strategic assessment of your polo neck situation: do they make you look too top heavy? If petite and big busted, always layer something on top to break up the upper body. If more curvaceous, avoid altogether and go for low scoop- or V-necks instead.

Boy/Straight (tall and lacking in curves):

✦ Having a tall, slim figure is the perfect backdrop for the military look so make a statement with bold decorative detailing on jackets.

✦ Watch the shape of combat trousers and make sure they are not too loose around the bottom and thighs as they will swamp you.

✦ Always accessorise jackets with a wide belt to create curves.

Strawberry Shaped
(broad shoulders and a wide back):

✦ Don't wear shirts buttoned too high and avoid epaulettes as these will square off your shoulders.

✦ Balance out upper and lower body differences by going for wider cut trousers rather than slim-leg styles.

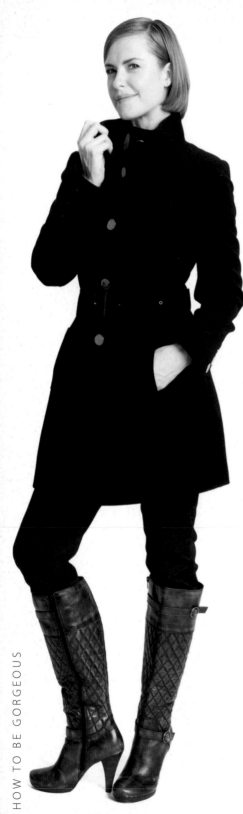

Seasoning

AS I SAY, BEFORE YOU WRITE OFF
THIS STYLE AS A WINTER LOOK,
remember that in the summer you can
swap the heavy wools and dark sombre
colours for lighter tones in cool crisp
cottons and linens. Nautical & Safari
trends are perfect for creating a capsule
wardrobe that is an essential part of any
TOP GUN goddess' all-weather kit:

Spring/Summer

1. SAFARI JACKET
2. SHIRT DRESS
3. TAILORED SHORTS
4. ANIMAL PRINT
5. VESTS (in khaki and white)
6. COTTON BLAZER
7. BOAT-NECK T-SHIRT
8. WHITE COTTON SKIRT

Autumn/Winter

1. LONG-SLEEVED STRIPED TOP
2. MILITARY-STYLE WINTER COAT
3. NAVY WIDE-LEG TROUSERS
4. HEAVY WOOLLEN CAPE
5. WELLINGTON BOOTS
6. LEATHER AVIATOR JACKET

RECIPE FOR *Success*

YOU DON'T HAVE TO BE G.I. JANE TO MAKE THE TOP GUN LOOK WORK FOR YOUR LIFESTYLE. Put together in the right way, it can be worn day or night, for any occasion.

1. School Run

For effortless, shipshape style, throw on a polo neck and Napoleon jacket with navy trousers and boots. If that still feels too dressed up you can always swap trousers for slim-leg jeans, or just throw on vest, combats, boots and a trench coat for completely easy chic. Beware of resorting to combats and trainers – this mismatch of Military and Sports Luxe won't win you any style medals!

2. The Office

For those of you who still need to look smart in the workplace but don't have to wear a suit, Military is a good halfway house. Mix and match military shirts and polo necks with long trousers and add an elasticated belt or a waistcoat for a little Forces flair.

3. The Early Evening Event

Once again Military is a good middle-of-the-road look; smart but with a fashionable edge. Wear jeans tucked into boots with a military-style shirt, waistcoat and belt around the waist. If the shirt still feels too formal, swap for vest or a cosy polo neck jumper.

Make-Up Masterclass

MILITARY-ESQUE MAKE-UP IS ALL ABOUT EDGE! IT'S ABOUT CREATING A LOOK THAT OOZES SEX APPEAL AND STRENGTH – making you a style force to be reckoned with! Win over any man with my expert beauty tactics.

1. Striking Eyes

Since your Military look has a touch of masculinity, it's vital that you show that you're all-woman by creating striking, sultry eyes.

✦ Using a sponge applicator, apply a shimmery, nude cream shadow to your entire eyelid, taking care to not go past the crease.

✦ Stroke a large eyeshadow brush along your natural eye socket to blend. Gently brush the eyeshadow colour up and out, focusing on the outer eyelid area.

✦ Completely line your upper and lower lids with dark slate-grey eyeliner. Stay as close as possible to your lash line and inner rims and smudge the line with a Q-tip.

✦ Apply a dark grey shadow along the line on your lower lids, smudging and softening the shadow as you do so. Apply a little dark grey shadow on the outer area of your lower eyelid and smudge.

2. Chiselled Cheeks

To give your look some serious edge, ditch pretty pink blush and instead chisel your cheekbones using a soft taupe hue.

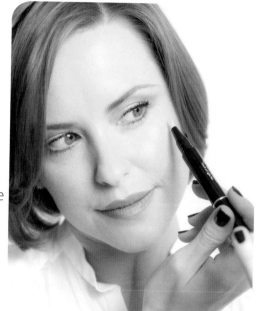

- ✦ Suck in your cheeks and lightly brush highlighter (or lightly coloured loose powder) just above the hollows of your cheeks, right back to your hairline.
- ✦ Still sucking in your cheeks, brush taupe-coloured blush along the the hollow of your cheeks.
- ✦ Lightly brush blush over the apples of your cheeks.
- ✦ Using a brush with thick bristles, lightly buff your cheeks so that the loose powder and blush lightly blend together, to create a more natural look.
- ✦ For a softer appearance, lightly sweep blush along your chin and on your temples.

3. Peachy Pout

Since your eyes are shouting all the command, keep lips simple. But, be sure to add a little sex appeal with a sweep of peach-tinted lip gloss to warm your complexion and complement your smoky eyes.

- ✦ Load lip gloss from the tube or pot onto a wand or make-up brush.
- ✦ Apply the gloss until the natural line of your lips has been filled.

Drop Dead Hair

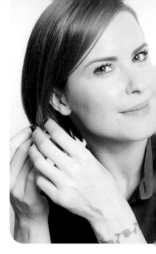

ERIN O'CONNOR IS FAMOUS FOR HER SHORT HAIR WHICH IS SEXY, SOPHISTICATED AND BOLD. Create your own statement with a hairstyle that sets off your Military style with real authority.

1. Bold Crop

Destroy the opposition and show off your beauty and confidence with a bold short crop. First check you have the right style for your hair type, to really push forward your advantage.

FINE HAIR

✦ **BOB IT.** One length or a slightly-layered bob work well with fine hair as these cuts make the hair appear thicker – especially if it already has a bit of natural wave.

✦ **PICK A PIXIE.** Short pixie-like cuts with lots of texture and layers can work well for fine hair. Just use plenty of mousse or gel to keep it messy-looking.

MEDIUM HAIR

✦ **PLAY UP THE CURL.** If your hair has curl to it, don't fight it. Short layered bobs with scrunched-in curls look great and are easy to style.

✦   **FLIP OUT.** Medium hair types are perfect for hairstyles that flip at the ends. Try a chin-length number or slightly longer bob with razored ends for head-turning Military chic.

THICK HAIR

✦   **KEEP IT SIMPLE.** A busy urban warrior doesn't have much time for styling their hair, so why not try keeping it simple with a sleek bob? This works best on straight hair and is super-easy to style. Update this look by having the ends razored to soften the style and add movement.

2. Statement Fringe

Nothing updates an old hairstyle more than adding a statement fringe. Bold fringes will frame your eyes and give you instant **Top Gun** style icon status. Check which fringe is best for you.

✦   Square-shaped faces suit a long, wispy layered fringe. Add a few small layers to the front of your face to soften the edges, giving you a more rounded look.

✦   Oval-shaped faces suit any length, shape or heaviness of fringe. An oval face is very versatile, so you can have fun experimenting with different styles.

✦   Heart-shaped faces suit a blunt, heavy fringe that will soften the chin and make the face appear more in proportion.

✦   Long, pointy faces suit a side fringe that is gently angled to soften the face shape.

✦   Round-shaped faces suit a soft, layered fringe that is slightly angled to the side to add a bit of length to the face.

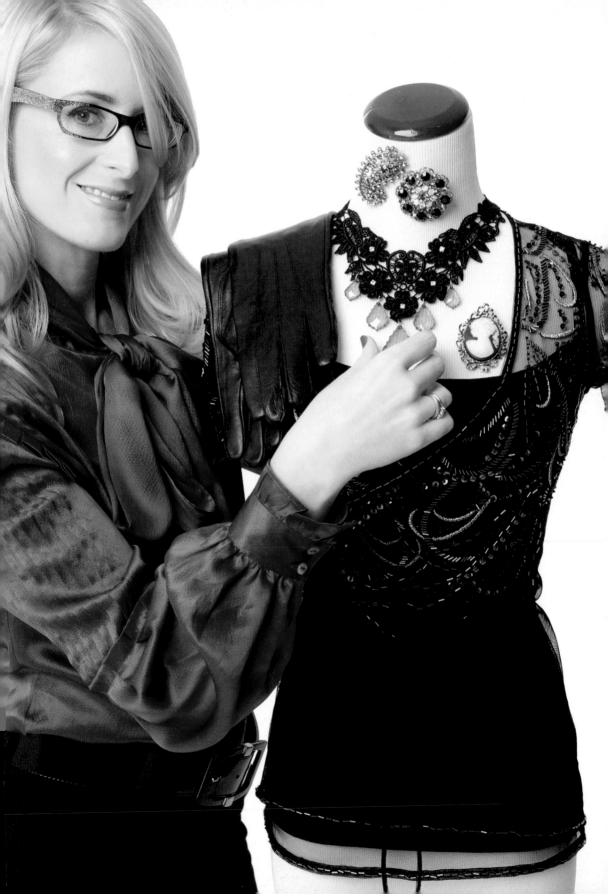

chapter 9

Victoriana

IF ONE IS NOT AMUSED BY MODERN FASHION, TRY
VICTORIANA: A VINTAGE STYLE FIT FOR A QUEEN.

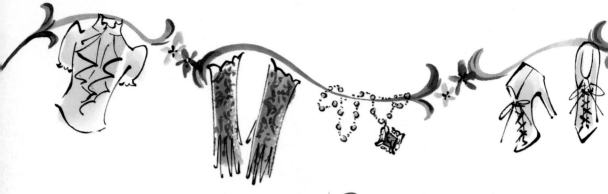

VICTORIA'S *Secret*

FOR 64 YEARS QUEEN VICTORIA REIGNED OVER THE BRITISH EMPIRE . . .
AND OVER THE VICTORIAN FASHION ELITE TOO. When she went
into mourning after the death of her husband the nation followed suit,
and dark, dreamy gothic style was born. Now, over 100 years later,
diehard fashionistas go back to black whenever they want effortless chic.

Inspiration FROM THE A-LIST

ONCE THE ETERNAL ROCK CHICK, THE NATION HAS WATCHED TEAR-
AWAY TEEN, KELLY OSBOURNE GROW INTO A SOPHISTICATED YOUNG
WOMAN, WITH A DRESS SENSE TO MATCH. Although black is still best
with Kelly, the oversized band T-shirts have been replaced by figure-hugging
gothic dresses which show off her womanly form in all its glory.

Designers have flocked to lace her into all sorts of fabulous structured outfits
that manipulate and show off her curvaceous figure. But what makes Kelly's
take on Victoriana all the more appealing is the way she mismatches period-

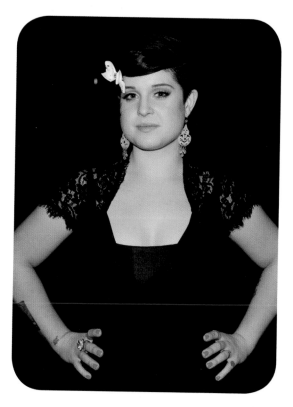

'I LOVE DOING MY OWN THING WITH FASHION. EVEN THOUGH BLACK IS MOST DEFINITELY MY FAVOURITE COLOUR, I AM ALWAYS MIXING AND MATCHING STYLES FROM DIFFERENT PERIODS IN TIME THAT SHOW OFF AND FLATTER MY CURVES. '

Kelly Osbourne

influenced pieces and vamps them up with modern-day items. Delicate lace or crochet dresses teamed with bright, stacked patent heels and chainmail bags are the hallmarks of Kelly's style, especially when worn with dark painted lips and nails. Likewise her day look is always the perfect balance of costume drama and contemporary glamour: high-collared frilled blouses with fitted leather jackets, black jeans and heavy boots.

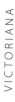

Key INGREDIENTS

THE VICTORIANA LOOK SPANS 64 YEARS OF FASHION, FROM THE BRIGHT AND FLAMBOYANT TO THE DARK AND DECADENT. However you want to work this style, the one important factor is the well-defined waist – so be prepared to cinch yourself in for an ultra-feminine silhouette! Here are the key ingredients you need to add a Victorian twist to your wardrobe.

1 THE HIGH-NECK FRILLED BLOUSE

This is the one essential piece for anyone looking to recreate this look. Victoriana **BLOUSES** should be in black, grey, white or cream with piecrust collars (high-neck collar with a frill around the edge) and neat little frills on shoulders, running down the centre of the blouse and/or around the edges of cuffs. Sleeves can be capped or puffed, for maximum authenticity. These blouses look best when contrasted against a sharp, tailored jacket to create the perfect balance between femininity and strength.

2 THE FITTED LEATHER JACKET

This is the modern-day version of the Victorian jacket. Extremely fitted against the body, it should sit just above hips. Shoulders should have a little puff detail to add femininity. Keep zip fastenings small or concealed to avoid a Rock Chick style.

Tip *Don't just stick with black; shades of tan, grey and deep red can add vibrancy to the look and stop it looking so dark.*

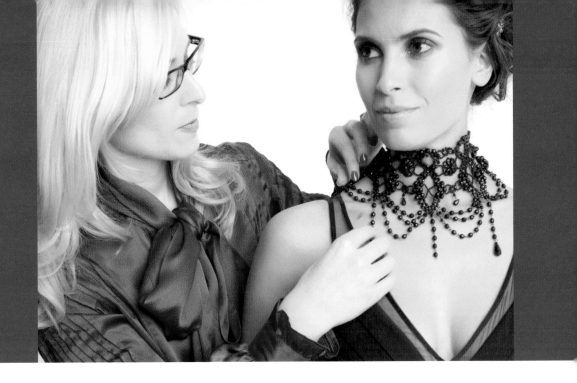

3 DRAMATIC BLACK DRESS

To give the traditional Victorian DRESS a new-Millennium twist, opt for a knee-length version in a style that suits you. Keep it simple or try one with beading, sheer detailing or even tiers and flounces. Wear with black tights for full gothic effect.

> *Tip* *BLACK DRESSES are gorgeously flattering. If you have a slim figure go for a fitted style to show off your shape. If on the other hand you are conscious of your lower body, a full skirt can hide a multitude of sins. Make sure to add big detailed jewellery.*

4 DISTRESSED JEANS

JEANS help to soften this austere look, especially if they're faded or distressed. Pick and choose between shades of blues, greys and blacks. Team with vintage lace blouses and lace-up boots to encapsulate the mood without overloading on nostalgia.

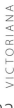

5 BLACK EMBELLISHED TOP

For a touch of daytime drama or a chance to really vamp it up for the evening, **BLACK TOPS** adorned with jet beading, lace, crochet, ribbons and fringing are perfect. Tops should be fitted and detail should be focused around the neckline, then choose between long puffed sleeves or little capped styles.

> *Tip*
> *Be careful not to overdo the embellishment. Too much lace, crochet and fringing can be a little Miss Havisham. Layer underneath a fitted jacket or suit if you're at all uncertain.*

6 CHIFFON RUFFLED BLOUSE

A **CHIFFON RUFFLED BLOUSE** in a vibrant colour will help soften this look. For a true Victoriana vibe keep the ruffles small and delicate.

7 TULIP-SHAPED SKIRT

Great for emphasising small waists, the shorter, far more functional **TULIP SKIRT** is the contemporary version of heavy nineteenth-century skirts. Wear just above the knee and team with fitted tops (tucked in to show off your waist), black tights and lace-up boots. Tulip-shaped skirts are a great way to disguise chunky calves and thighs, – the extra volume adds width creating the illusion of slimmer pins.

8 CORSET

CORSETS always have their place on the catwalk, and are easier to wear than you think. For day, simple cotton ones can be worn layered over a shirt, blouse or T-shirt; for a more dramatic evening look wear on its own in black satin or layered lace. The key is to create that nipped-in waist effect, irrespective of your shape or size. Stick with dark shades to let your inner goth rule!

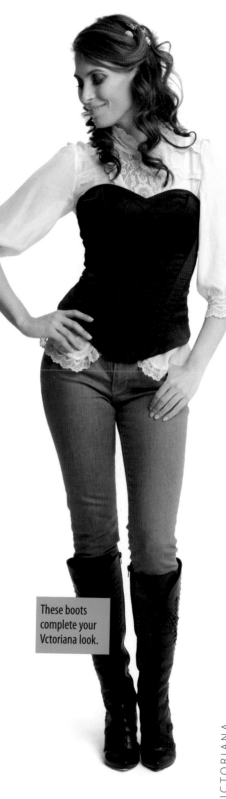

> *Tip* *Beware of the dreaded muffin top. Always wear high-rise jeans, trousers or skirts to avoid any really embarrassing overspill!*

9 VELVET BLAZER

Add a touch of Victorian luxury to the most pared-down outfit. A tailored VELVET BLAZER teamed with jeans perfectly combines sophistication with a fashionable edge. Deep purple, emerald, or midnight blue will add colour without detracting from the overall look.

10 LACE-UP BOOTS

Choose between knee-length, calf or ankle boots and decide whether a pointed or round toe suits you best. Go for black or rich dark colours such as deep purple as these will integrate more easily with the rest of the look.

These boots complete your Vctoriana look.

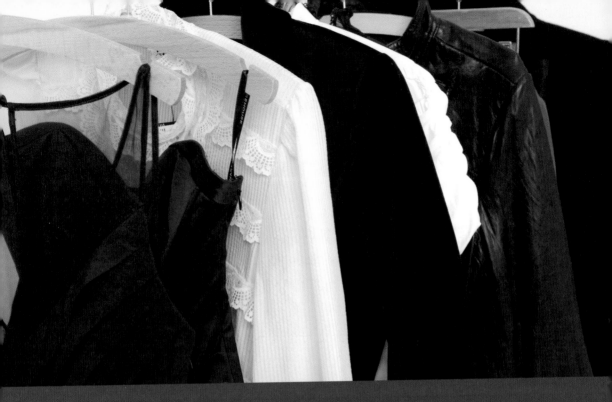

Trimmings

VICTORIAN FASHION WAS COVERED IN FINE DETAILING AND EMBELLISHMENT, and this trend also extended to the accessories they used to complement their look. Many pieces are still popular accessory choices today, so go raid that high street!

✦ JET BEADED CHOKER/NECKLACE

Highly ornate, large CHOKER-STYLE NECKLACES make the simplest of outfits look decadent. Made originally from black jet, these days plastic equivalents will also do the trick. If you don't want to draw attention to your neck, invest in a few strings of jet beads of varying lengths to create the same vampish effect.

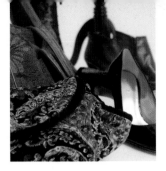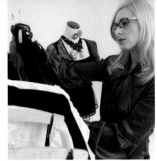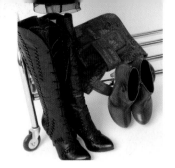

✦ CAMEO BROOCH

No self-respecting Victorian vixen would go out without a CAMEO brooch pinned to her blouse or jacket. The best are original vintage ones, but high street copies can be just as good and are easy to source. For a more modern twist wear a cluster of cameos and other brooches together.

✦ EMBELLISHED PURSE

Leave the old clutch bag at home and instead opt for pretty embroidered or beaded PURSE to hold your pennies on a ladylike evening out.

✦ TAPESTRY HANDBAGS

A great opportunity for adding a bit of colour to the sometimes dark, sombre outfits of this era. Mary-Poppins-style handbags were all the rage back then, and are now the perfect day bag for carrying everything in.

✦ LACE TRIM ACCESSORIES

Delicate cuffs, or pretty detachable collars; a little LACE always adds a touch of period drama to any outfit – but too much can look stuffy. Lace-printed plastic bracelets will add a more modern flair.

✦ BOOTIES

Alongside the lace-up boots, low ankle boots with button detailing up the side of the shoe are a great leg-lengthening alternative when wearing skirts and dresses.

✦ LONG LEATHER GLOVES

For real gothic influence and to add a touch of mystique to your look, invest in a pair of long or ¾-length black leather GLOVES.

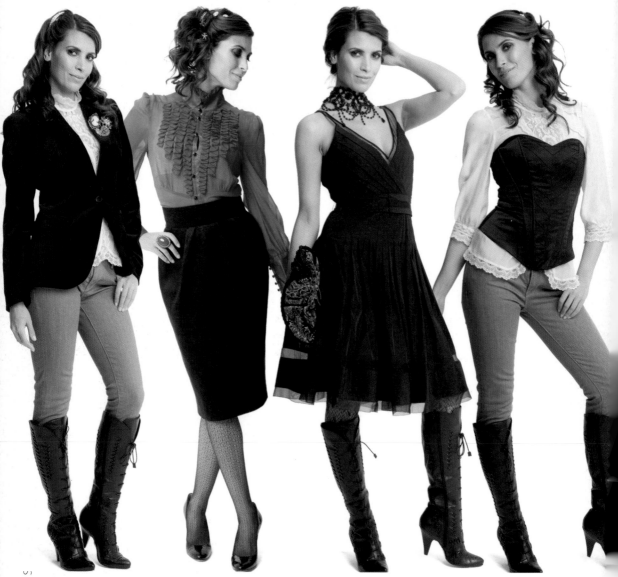

✦ The velvet jacket + lace-up boots + high-necked blouse

✦ The high-necked blouse + tulip-shaped skirt

✦ The A-line dress + choker necklace + tapestry bag

✦ The chiffon blouse + corset + lace-up boots

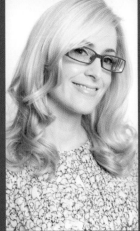

Styling
SUGGESTIONS

	HIGH-NECKED FRILLED BLOUSE	DISTRESSED JEANS	LEATHER JACKET	BLACK EMBELLISHED TOP	PRINCESS/A-LINE DRESS	CHIFFON RUFFLED BLOUSE	TULIP-SHAPED SKIRT	CORSET	VELVET JACKET	*Now...* ACCESSORISE YOUR OUTFIT
1	✓	✓	✓							LACE-UP BOOTS AND TAPESTRY BAG
2		✓				✓			✓	LACE-UP BOOTS OR BOOTIES, CAMEO BROOCH, COIN PURSE
3			✓	✓			✓			BOOTIES, BLACK TIGHTS AND TAPESTRY BAG
4					✓				✓	LACE-UP BOOTS, BLACK TIGHTS, BROOCHES AND EITHER CHOKER OR LONG JET BEADS
5		✓						✓	✓	BOOTIES, CHOKER AND COIN PURSE
6	✓						✓			LACE-UP BOOTS AND CAMEO BROOCH
7			✓		✓					LACE-UP BOOTS OR BOOTIES, BLACK TIGHTS, LONG JET BEADS
8						✓	✓		✓	BOOTIES, BLACK TIGHTS, CLUSTER OF CAMEO BROOCHES
9			✓				✓	✓		LACE-UP BOOTS, BLACK TIGHTS, COIN PURSE AND LEATHER GLOVES
10		✓	✓	✓						LACE-UP BOOTS, LACE CUFF, AND TAPESTRY BAG

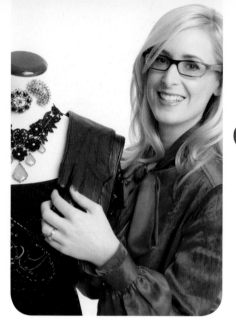

Wear it
YOUR WAY

IF QUEEN VICTORIA COULD PULL THIS
LOOK OFF, SO CAN YOU! Here are some
tips on how to get it right for you:

Pear Shapes
(carry weight on their hips and bum):

✦ When it comes to corsets, Pears need to watch the bottom line.
   Longer styles that sit over the hips are great, and even better still are
   typical Victorian shapes that dip forward at the front and back,
   creating the illusion of leaner torso and slimmer hips.
✦ Choker necklaces are ideal as they will draw attention upwards
   towards your slim neck and chest.

Apple Shapes
(carry weight on their tummy and chest):

✦ Make sure frills and ruffles on blouses run vertically down the body in
   order to streamline your figure.
✦ Tulip-shaped skirts can exaggerate round tummies, so swap for a
   wide-waistband skirt with bustle detail at the back to balance out
   the silhouette.

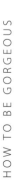
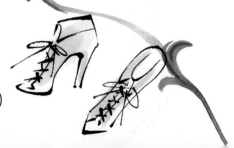

Hourglass
(curvaceous all over with a small waist):

✦ With high-neck Victoriana blouses make sure you leave a couple of buttons undone to give shape to the chest.

✦ Corsets are fantastic items for hourglass figures as they really define sexy curves – just make sure yours has a scalloped neckline and is high enough over the chest to give full support. You can always layer it under a tailored jacket or over a chiffon blouse for something more demure.

Boy/Straight *(tall and lacking in curves):*

✦ The tiers and flounces of Victoriana style dresses and tops are perfect for willowy frames. Go to town and really show off your figure by adding intricate embellishment into the mix.

✦ High-neck puff-sleeve Victoriana blouses can often look quite Headmistress-y on tall, slim frames. Avoid this by going for the more contemporary versions with capped sleeves that balance out proportions and show off your slim arms.

Strawberry Shaped
(broad shoulders and a wide back):

✦ Choker necklaces should be avoided if you've got broad shoulders. Instead opt for longer beaded styles, or vamp it up with cameo brooches worn on a chain.

✦ Always choose corsets that have a scalloped top edge for a super-flattering look.

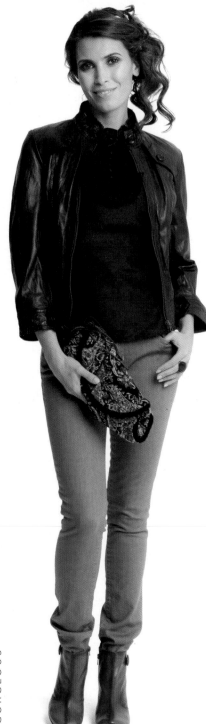

Seasoning

THE KEY TO VAMPING UP THE VICTORIANA LOOK is to always remember to mix and match together new and old fabrics, delicate lace and tougher, sexier fabrics. Get it right and it's a timeless look that you'll fall back on through the years and you'll never end up looking like an extra on a film set! Here are some extra pieces to help you work the look all year round:

Spring/Summer

1. WHITE COTTON SUNDRESS
2. FLOPPY STRAW HAT
3. LACE BLOUSE
4. DECK SHOES
5. PINSTRIPED COTTON JACKET
6. FLOATY FLORAL SKIRT
7. PRINCESS-LINE FLORAL DRESS

Autumn/Winter

1. FUR MUFF
2. WHITE LACE-UP BOOTS
3. WOOLLEN CAPE
4. LONG BLACK SKIRT
5. DARK-COLOURED SHAWL
6. VELVET BOLERO

RECIPE FOR *Success*

SOME ELEMENTS OF THE LOOK ARE BEST RESERVED FOR THE WEEKEND (that bustle might get in the way at work!) but there are easy outfits you can use to vamp up your wardrobe in a very subtle way.

1. Day to Dinner

Victoriana is the perfect look for not being too dressy during the day or too under-dressed for the evening. Team a black embellished top with distressed jeans and add leather jacket and lace-up boots. For a more elegant look swap the leather jacket for a velvet blazer in a deep vibrant colour.

2. Trendy Cocktail bar

A Victorian corset is a must for the weekends – so dress up, feel ultra-feminine and be prepared for lots of attention! Simply wear with distressed jeans, lace-up boots and a beaded choker, or a little bolero to cover the tops of your arms.

3. Night at the Theatre

A dramatic event needs a dramatic outfit! Choose between a princess-line dress or tulip skirt and frilled blouse, with black tights and booties. Finish off the whole look with a leather jacket to see you from the car to Dress Circle.

4. Hot Date

Go for a corset to show your date you're all woman! Pair with either jeans or a tulip skirt and add a leather jacket, black beaded choker and booties. If you're worried about being too full-on (or not enjoying your dinner!) then go for an embellished dress with booties and a soft velvet jacket.

FINISHING TOUCHES

Make-Up Masterclass

BY DAY THE VICTORIANA LOOK IS SUBDUED, SUBTLE AND FLUSHED; after hours, it's sexy, dark and glam! Here's how to take this look from day to night.

1. Ladylike Luxe

Swap dewy or illuminating foundations and concealers for creamy, matt products and keep shine at bay throughout the day with a vintage 'oh so pretty' nose-powdering compact. This is one make-up item you'll be happy to apply in public!

✦ While bronzer is a big no for this look, blush is essential to bring your vintage complexion to life.

✦ Choose a pretty pink blush; the deeper pink your skin tone, the deeper pink you can afford to go. But keep it natural not theatrical.

2. Dawn to Dusk Eyes

DAY

✦ Apply a light layer of foundation to your eyes to create a perfect base, allow a few seconds to dry and dust with loose powder.

- Next, sweep a bone or ivory coloured matt eyeshadow across the lower lid.
- Awaken your eyes by highlighting them with an irridescent pearl eye shadow. Dab a Q-tip into the shadow and apply lightly to the inner corners of both eyes.
- Enhance each individual lash with a couple of sweeps of lash-separating mascara to your top and bottom lashes.

NIGHT

- Keep your basic make-up the same, but now add lots of smudgy kohl and just a touch of dark eyeshadow.
- Lightly apply the kohl on the inside of the lower lid. The eyeliner on the lower lid will transfer to the upper lid as you blink. If your eyes are small, only apply liner along the top lid.
- Now apply kohl pencil to the top lash line, getting the colour as close to the lashes as possible.
- Carefully apply eyeshadow of the same colour over the kohl on the top lid with a Q-tip, smudging the line as you go, to soften the effect. You don't want any harsh lines.
- With the remains of the eyeshadow on your Q-tip, smudge a little colour under the lower lash line a quarter of the way in.
- Lastly dab a little of the pearl irridescent eyeshadow onto your brow bone and blend with your ring finger.

Drop Dead Hair

THE EXPRESSION, 'A WOMAN'S CROWNING GLORY' dates back to the Victorian period when waves, coquettish curls, and plaits were becomingly arranged and adorned with jewel-embellished hair pins and bows. In Victorian times a woman's hair was very important to her overall image.

Shoot forward 100 years and that's still very much the case. KELLY OSBOURNE is a perfect example of a modern-day vamp; her love affair with scissors and dye appears to be never-ending. Short, long, black or blonde – her hair always makes her stand out from the fashion pack. You don't have to be as brave as Ms Osbourne to finish off your Victoriana look in style. Just take a tip from history with these easy vintage hair trends:

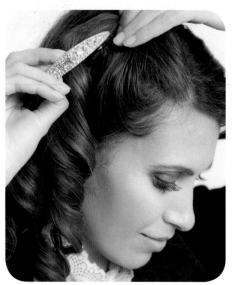

1. Hair Jewellery

Whether your hair is long or short, dark or blonde, curly or straight, every Victoriana fashionista must own a selection of embellished hair clips, grips, pins and forks.

✦ Hair accessories with a yesteryear vibe are worth their weight in gold! Seek out clips adorned with faux rubies, diamonds, pearls, sapphires and onyx stones to add some retro bling to your locks.

- ✦ Give plain metal clips an overhaul by affixing buttons, gems, felt designs, patches and small silk flowers to the ends with liquid glue or adhesive dots.
- ✦ Add short ribbon ties to the edges of the hair clips or use a single bow for a touch of colour.

2. Vintage Rags

This simple up-do looks gorgeous on curly hair. If your hair is straight why not try curling it using hot tongs?

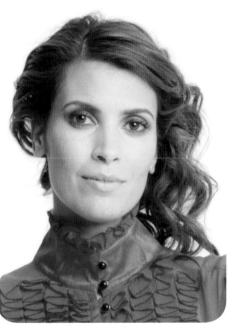

- ✦ Wash your hair and condition it as you normally would. Use a comb to remove the tangles and allow it to dry almost completely.
- ✦ Separate your hair into sections and curl each section using hot tongs.
- ✦ Then roll each curl up and pin to allow the curl to set while curling the rest of your hair.
- ✦ Once finished, remove all of the pins and use your fingers to lightly comb through your hair.
- ✦ To complete this look, gather up your curls an inch or so above the nape of your neck and secure loosely with a vintage-looking claw clip.
- ✦ Leave curl tendrils loose on the sides and in the fringe area to soften the look around your face.

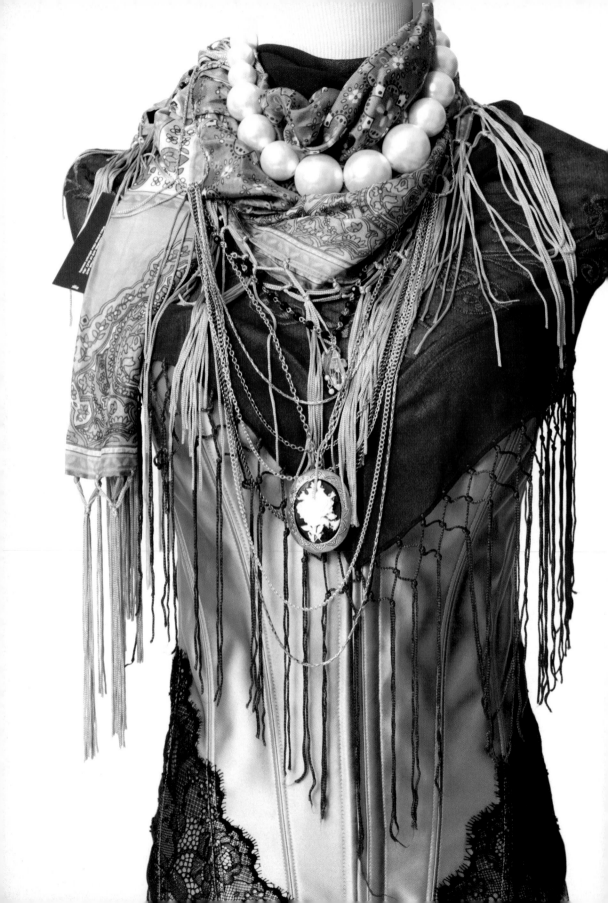

chapter 10

Romantic

THERE'S NOTHING LIKE A LITTLE ROMANCE TO MAKE
A GIRL FEEL ULTRA-FEMININE, SO WHY NOT START A
REAL LOVE AFFAIR WITH THIS GORGEOUS STYLE?

‘A LADY'S IMAGINATION IS VERY RAPID; IT JUMPS FROM ADMIRATION TO LOVE, FROM LOVE TO MATRIMONY, IN A MOMENT.’

Jane Austen, Pride and Prejudice

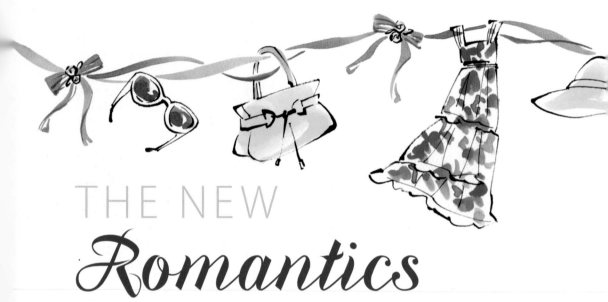

THE NEW
Romantics

IN THE 1980S, DRESSING UP FOR BOTH DAY AND NIGHT BECAME THE NORM. The New Romantics experimented with a flamboyant and dramatic sense of dress that looked back in history, and adopted the decadent fabrics and intricate adornment of Austen's heroes and heroines. Designers like Vivienne Westwood gave clothes a theatrical twist with luscious details like beading, lace, satin appliqué and layers of tiers and ruffles. Underwear became the new outwear, with pretty camisoles under soft cashmere cardigans emerging as a staple look for any fashion conscious ROMANTIC.

Inspiration
FROM THE A-LIST

ALWAYS SEEN IN FLOATY FULL-LENGTH GOWNS ON THE RED CARPET, KEIRA KNIGHTLEY mixes old Hollywood glamour with classic refined elegance. Plunging necklines, barely covered shoulders, sumptuous fabrics in the softest hues all make up the elements of a modern fairytale romance.

Off-duty, Keira continues her whimsical style by blending elements of the theatre, ballet studio and boudoir together to create unusual, charming looks. Her boyish frame is feminised in frilly pirate shirts with high-waist trousers, pretty floral tea dresses with soft buttery leather jackets and delicate antique-looking camis layered under soft, cosy knits. Day or night, her relaxed off-beat style proves that romantic fashions are not just reserved for girly girls – they can be worn by anyone. For knockout romance, beautiful floor-sweeping gowns are the ultimate outfit for any girl looking to be swept off her feet by the man of her dreams.

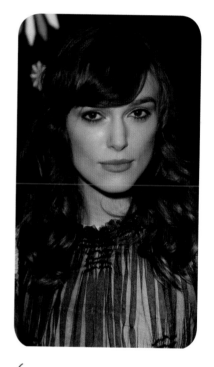

'I THINK EVERY GIRL IS LOOKING FOR HER MR DARCY.'

Keira Knightley

Key INGREDIENTS

MODERN-DAY ROMANCE IS NOT JUST ABOUT LOOKING PRETTY; it's about celebrating femininity, mixing together styles and influences. Theatre, ballet, film and novels all play their role in creating femme fatale fashion. These key pieces will add some flirtatious fun to your wardrobe.

1 MAXI DRESS

Sadly for most of us there is not much requirement for show-stopping, floor-sweeping gowns, but MAXI DRESSES in light layers of chiffon, tulle and silk jersey mean you can bring a touch of romance to any day of the week. Tone down further by going for a style with a large, swirly print. Maxi dresses can overwhelm a slim, petite figure and make a larger person look dumpy. Team with a belt to create shape, and always wear heels.

2 FLIPPY SKIRT

Flounces, tiers or full circular shapes in layers of chiffon add extra oomph and are a modern take on the ballerina's tutu. The complete antithesis of the rigid pencil skirt, these tend to flip up in the back whenever there's a brisk wind or you've got to run for a bus. Choose between pretty floral prints or delicate detailing.

3 CAMISOLE

Silks and satins in bright, jewel colours or soft, pinky tones with delicate lace trim detail – underwear this pretty shouldn't be hidden! CAMISOLES are something every woman can wear whatever their age, size or shape. Why not source from a vintage shop to add a little vintage elegance?

4 FLIRTY TEA DRESS

Unlike the full maxi dress, the TEA DRESS can be fitted or cut on the bias with a high or low neckline. Ruffles, puffed sleeves, frilled hemlines, pin tucks and all things delicate can be piled on. Choose from small ditzy prints, big swirly patterns or bold colours – the choice is yours.

5 BODICE

The BODICE is less ornate than the corsets of the Victorian era. Avoid intricate detailing as the romantic version could look like exposed underwear. Keep it sculpted and simple in nudes or soft milky shades with moulded cups and panelled seams. For true romance, wear a bodice over a sheer chiffon blouse or tea dress. Best suited to women with smaller chests and slim waists.

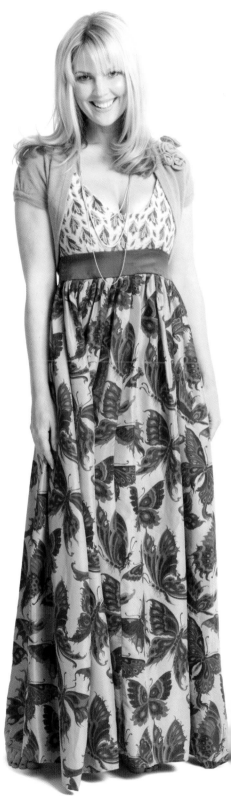

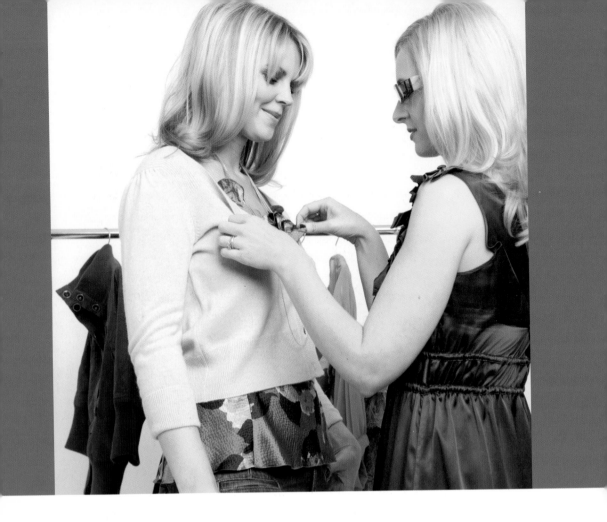

6 CASHMERE CARDIGAN

Make like a ballerina, and cover up in these soft, cosy little knitted cardigans that can be worn over chiffon blouses, camisoles or bodices. Go for soft, washed-out shades: powder blue, mint, cream or violet. If your budget won't stretch to cashmere, wool and acrylic mixes are perfect.

7 LEATHER JACKET

Unlike all the other leather jackets mentioned in this book, a romantic LEATHER JACKET should be in the softest supple leather in nude colours. It toughens up the most delicate of outfits.

8 SHEER BLOUSE

Go for loose or fitted sleeved tops with abundance of ruffles or pin tuck detailing and big bows, or stick to simple tunic shapes with a vest in a contrasting colour layered underneath. Vibrant colours work just as well as pale muted tones.

Tip *Sheer blouses are über-feminine but can be quite draining on your skin tone. Always layer over a cami in a similar or a contrasting colour for a much more modern twist.*

9 PALE HIGH-WAIST JEANS

PALE BLUE or even WHITE JEANS are the perfect modern-day component to balance out all the wispy fabrics. The high waist enables voluminous tops to be tucked in, showing off feminine curves. Choose from flared or skinny varieties depending on the slimness of your legs. High-waisted jeans are a godsend for any women desperate to hide her post-baby belly. They're flattering for all ages, and help to define and accentuate the waist.

10 NUDE-COLOURED SHOES

With so many dainty styles floating around, NUDE- OR LIGHT TAN-COLOURED SHOES are essential footwear for lengthening your legs. Heels or flats work equally well; just remember to change to dark shoes if wearing dark tights. Make sure your shoes are at least one shade darker than your natural skin tone to create a contrast.

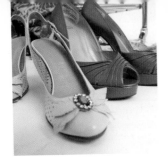
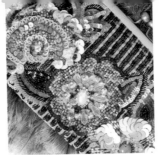
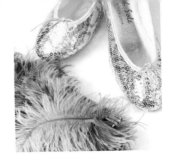

Trimmings

TO MY MIND, TRUE ROMANCE SHOULD BE EFFORTLESS AND EASY.
With that in mind, I've picked out a few fun accessories that will add
the finishing touches to this flirty look.

✦ PRETTY BRAS

Antique-coloured BRAS with ribbon and other pretty detailing are perfect
for layering under sheer blouses or peeking through dresses or camisoles,
for a little harmless flirtatious fun.

✦ VINTAGE LOOK PURSE

Ruffles, ribbons, lace or even stitched feather purses add a touch of
society-girl class to any outfit. Opt for authentic vintage for the real thing.

✦ EMBROIDERED SATCHEL

A heavy leather bag is overkill with this look, but an embroidered
SATCHEL in either tan leather, suede or fabric is a good compromise. That
way you can maintain the romance and will still be able to carry around
all your worldly possessions.

✦ FRINGED SCARF

Try a lace, silk or organza SCARF in pretty washed-out tones. Wear
draped over shoulders, wrapped around your neck or even
looped through your jeans to create an unusual belt.

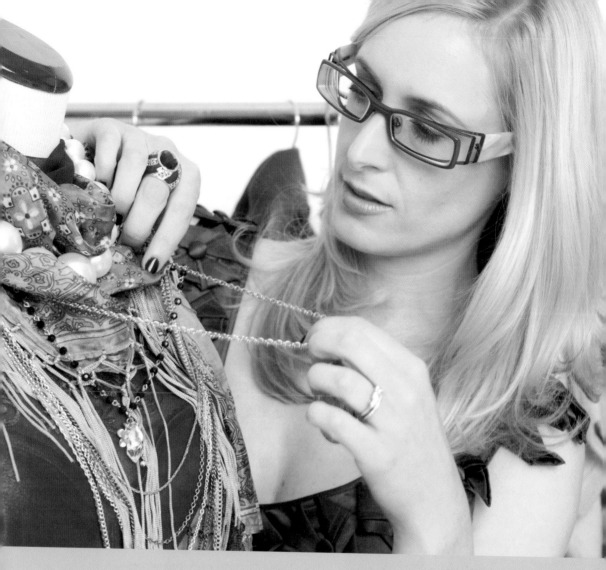

✦ THEATRICAL JEWELS

Big over-sized pearls layered together in various lengths work the thespian look. Alternatively, jewelled chokers and chandelier earrings in bright-coloured stones add a touch of period drama.

✦ LONG, GOLD CHAINS

Long, delicate GOLD CHAINS or filigree bangles are great, but even small gold hoops can help finish off the Romantic look.

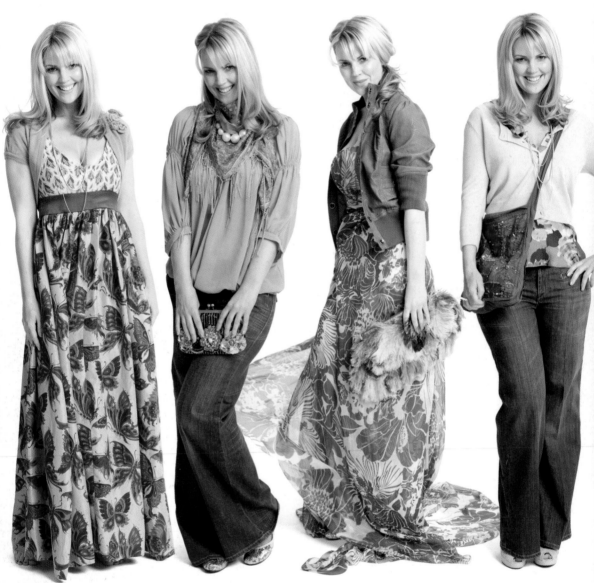

✦ The maxi dress + cashmere cardigan + gold necklaces

✦ The sheer blouse + fringed scarf + jewelled flats

✦ The maxi dress + leather jacket + nude flats

✦ The cashmere cardigan + embroidered bag

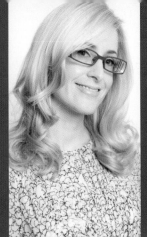

Styling SUGGESTIONS

Now... ACCESSORISE YOUR OUTFIT

	MAXI DRESS	CASHMERE CARDIGAN	FLIPPY SKIRT	CAMISOLE	BODICE	PALE JEANS	SHEER BLOUSE	TEA DRESS	LEATHER JACKET	Now... ACCESSORISE YOUR OUTFIT
1	✓	✓								HIPSTER BELT, NUDE HEELS AND LONG GOLD CHAINS
2		✓	✓		✓					SHOES OR CHUNKY BOOTS
3		✓		✓		✓				FRINGED SCARF, HEELS AND EMBROIDERED SATCHEL
4								✓	✓	THEATRICAL JEWELS OR SIMPLE GOLD NECKLACES, CHUNKY BOOTS
5					✓	✓	✓			NUDE HEELS
6	✓								✓	FRINGED SCARF
7		✓						✓		PRETTY BRA, GOLD BANGLES AND HEELS
8			✓	✓					✓	PRETTY BRA, THEATRICAL JEWELS
9			✓				✓		✓	HEELS AND EMBROIDERED BAG OR RUFFLED PURSE
10		✓	✓	✓						NUDE SHOES, LONG GOLD NECKLACES AND BANGLES

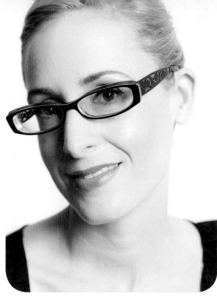

ℬ︎ear it
YOUR WAY

HERE ARE A FEW SIMPLE TIPS which I hope will enable you to fall in love with your wardrobe once again and marvel at the absolutely gorgeous curves you never knew you had:

Pear Shapes
(carry weight on their hips and bum):

✦ Watch tiers on skirts and dresses as they can highlight hips and bottom. However, a big ruffled hemline will draw the eye down and move attention away from your widest point.

✦ Avoid bias-cut dresses and skirts as fabric always emphasises the hips.

✦ Blouses with large ruffle detailing are ideal as they help draw attention upwards and away from your hips.

Apple Shapes
(carry weight on their tummy and chest):

✦ To avoid accentuating your tummy, don't go too high-waisted on jeans. The most flattering shapes have a wide waistband and sit just below the belly button.

✦ The maxi dress will always need a hipster belt to create the most slimming shape.

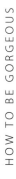

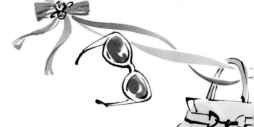

- Layering a fitted cami or vest top under a sheer blouse is an ideal way to create shape without wearing something too tight.

Hourglass
(curvaceous all over with a small waist):

- Always go for smaller-scale ruffles around bust area as big cascades can make you look very top-heavy.
- Since most hourglass shapes have bigger chests it's important that if bra straps are on show they don't resemble scaffolding! You could always do a DIY job on your favourite bra by attaching little ribbons and bows to dress the straps.

Boy/Straight *(tall and lacking in curves):*

- Layering a bodice over a voluminous top is an ideal way to inject curves and create shape.
- Very full skirts don't always suit straight shapes, so far better to go for a more A-line style with plenty of romantic tiers.

Strawberry Shaped
(broad shoulders and a wide back):

- Always stick with smaller ruffles on the upper half of the torso to avoid emphasising broadness.
- All jeans, skirts and dresses should be flared to balance out the proportions of lower and upper body.
- Soft, silk, low-cut camis layered under gorgeous knits are an ideal way to soften shoulders and break up the upper body.

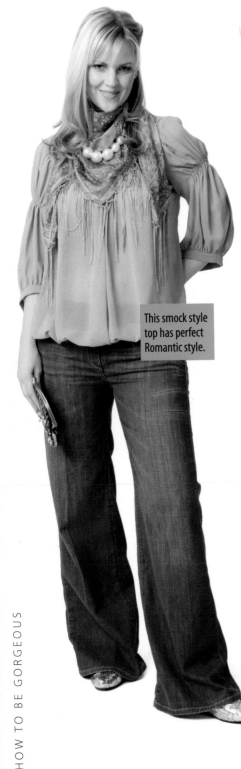

This smock style top has perfect Romantic style.

Seasoning

THE ROMANTIC LOOK IS OFTEN MORE OF A SUMMER STYLE due to the fine fabrics used. However, with some clever mixing, it can work for all seasons . . . which is no doubt a relief if you've already fallen head over heels in love with this look! Here are some seasonal extras you'll cherish:

Spring/Summer

1. FLORAL BLOUSES
2. SILK KIMONO TOP
3. HOT PANTS
4. BRODERIE ANGLAISE SMOCK TOP
5. RA-RA SKIRT
6. PALE DENIM JACKET/WAISTCOAT
7. CREAM COTTON BLAZER

Autumn/Winter

1. VIBRANTLY COLOURED RUFFLED SHIRTS
2. FAUX FUR STOLE
3. SOFT KNITTED BERET
4. THICK OVER-THE-KNEE SOCKS
5. LONG KNITTED SCARF
6. FISHTAIL WOOL SKIRT
7. RUFFLED/TIERED PARTY DRESS

RECIPE FOR *Success*

LIKE BOHO, ROMANTIC IS A LOOK THAT IS EASY TO DRESS UP OR DOWN WITH SIMPLE LAYERING. If you're a fan of the casual femininity of Boho daywear, you'll love the stylish softness of Romantic attire for the evening.

1. *Romantic Dinner*

Every girl loves to be romanced the good old-fashioned way (no matter what her age!) and always needs a fool-proof outfit should an invitation come her way. A pretty tea dress teamed with a little cardigan and perhaps a naughty flash of a pretty bra will definitely leave him wanting more!

2. *Black Tie Event*

Although these events don't come along all that often, when they do you should be ready to bring out your full-length gown. Go for a style in a plain, luxurious fabric for classic timeless elegance. Drape a fringed scarf around shoulders and accessorise with gold jewellery and ruffled bag.

3. *Day Out with Friends*

Want to make an effort without looking like you tried? If so, a tea dress toned down with leather jacket and boots is a very modern look. For something less edgy, jeans and a sheer blouse or a flippy skirt, little vest and cashmere cardigan will look effortlessly gorgeous too.

4. *Garden Party*

Garden parties and barbeques create the perfect setting for light-hearted flirtation. A maxi dress in swirly floral prints teamed either with cardigan or fringed scarf is an easy relaxed look for long, hot summer nights.

FINISHING TOUCHES
Make-Up Masterclass

He loves me, he loves me not? Grab the attention of your Mr. Darcy with Romantic make-up in light shimmers and soft, smoky shadows, and highlight your best features without overpowering your looks. Follow my simple steps and rekindle your love-affair with make-up all over again.

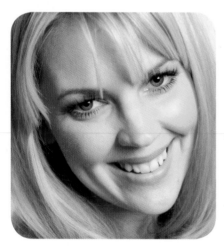

1. Irridescent Foundation

For a light, fresh and luminous effect use a light moisturiser to prime your face before you start.

+ With clean hands, mix one part irridescent face cream into two parts liquid foundation. Blend well.
+ Follow with a little concealer under the eyes and again, blend well.

2. Blush of Innocents

Complement your complexion with the softest hue of cream blush to give a truly innocent flush to your cheeks.

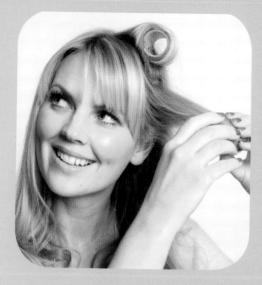

Drop Dead Hair

ROMANTIC HAIR IS HEALTHY, TOUCHABLE AND SEXY! Get the Romantic look and treat your tresses as your finest fashion accessory yet.

1. Wavy, Long Heroine Hair

- Blow-dry the ends of your hair under to create movement.
- Separate your hair into sections.
- With a curling iron, starting at the front of your head, wrap 2-3 inch sections of hair around the curling iron, bottom to top (the more hair you wrap around the iron the less curl you will achieve) to create loose waves as opposed to tight curls. Hold the hair around the iron for 15 to 20 seconds.
- Repeat for each section of your hair.
- Shake your head gently or tug on the curls a bit to create a looser Romantic look.

> **Tip** *Adding a pretty accessory to short to mid-length hair is a sure-fire way to set hearts a-fluttering.*

Get Gorgeous...

BEAUTY ESSENTIALS

NOW YOUR WARDROBE'S FULL OF BEAUTIFUL, VERSATILE OUTFITS IT'S TIME TO SHOP FOR THE ULTIMATE HAIR AND MAKE-UP PRODUCTS.

These are THE products. I've divided them into DAY and NIGHT categories – but really it's all about what works for you and your lifestyle. Don't forget to consult each chapter's FINISHING TOUCHES section to match your hair and make-up to your overall look.

SKIN

Day

- ✦ **Cream foundation:** Max Factor Flawless Perfection
- ✦ **Tinted moisturiser:** Body Shop Moisture Foundation SPF 15
- ✦ **Cream concealer:** Rimmel London Recover Concealer
- ✦ **Matt primer:** Body Shop Colourings, Matte It Face & Lips

Night

- ✦ **Mineral foundation:** bareMinerals SPF 15
- ✦ **Illuminating primer:** Boots No.7 High Lights Illuminating Lotion
- ✦ **Highlighter pen:** Boots No.7 Instant Radiance Concealer Pen
- ✦ **Cream highlighter:** Barry M Shimmer Cream

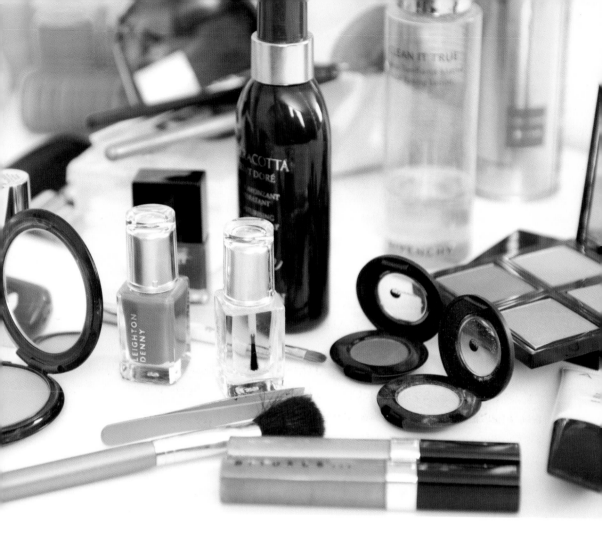

CHEEKS

Day

✦ **Cream blush**: Revlon Cream Blush
✦ **Sheer blush**: Benefit Benetint

Night

✦ **Powder blush:** Body Shop Colourings
✦ **Face/cheek shimmer:** Maybelline Dream Sunglow
Instant Shimmer

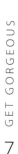

EYES

Day

- ✦ **Eyebrow pencil:** Maybelline Eyebrow Pencil
- ✦ **Mascara:** Max Factor Masterpiece Max
- ✦ **Eyeshadow palette:** GOSH Quattro Eyeshadow Palette in Goldfinger
- ✦ **Eyeliner pencil:** GOSH Kohl Eye Pencil

Night

- ✦ **Eyelash curlers:** Body Shop Eyelash Curlers
- ✦ **Metallic eyeshadow:** L'Oreal Colour Appeal Platinum Eyeshadow
- ✦ **Liquid eyeliner:** Collection 2000 Fast Stroke Liquid Eyeliner

LIPS

Day

- ✦ **Transparent gloss:** Max Factor Silk Gloss in Crystal Dew
- ✦ **Sheer lipstick:** Revlon Super Lustrous Shiny Sheers in red
- ✦ **Nude lipstick:** L'Oreal Colour Riche Made For Me Naturals

Night

- ✦ **Irridescent gloss:** Boots Natural Collection in Toffee Cream
- ✦ **Red lipstick:** Maybelline Superstay 18 Hour Wear Lipstick in Red
- ✦ **Lip-pumping gloss:** DuWop Lip Venom in Pink Shimmer

HAIR

Day

- ✦ **Wax/pomade/putty:** Dax Short and Neat Wax
- ✦ **Volumiser:** Andrew Collinge Weightless Volume Protection
- ✦ **Anti-frizz:** Redken Smooth/John Frieda Frizz Ease

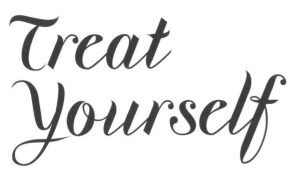

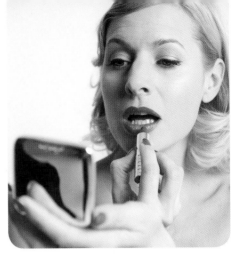

Treat Yourself

NOTHING MAKES YOU FEEL GORGEOUS LIKE LUXURIOUS MAKE-UP AND HAIR PRODUCTS, so why not finish off your look with these A-list treats?

MAKE-UP

✦ **Illuminating primer:** MAC Strobe Cream
✦ **Face/cheek shimmer:** Bobbi Brown Shimmer Brick
✦ **Eyelash curlers:** She Uemura Eyelash Curlers
✦ **Metallic eyeshadow:** MAC Pigment Eyeshadow in Gold
✦ **Lip gloss:** Estée Lauder 01 Quartz
✦ **Highlighter pen:** YSL Touche Éclat
✦ **Powder blush:** Stila Cheek Colour
✦ **Volumising mascara:** Christian Dior DiorShow Mascara
✦ **Eyeliner:** Clinique Eye Defining Liquid Liner
✦ **Lipstick:** Bobbi Brown Pale Pink 21

HAIR

✦ **Hair putty:** Fudge Hair Shaper
✦ **Volumiser:** Kerastase Mousse Volumactive
✦ **Anti-frizz spray:** Bumble and Bumble Defrizz
✦ **Styling cream:** American Crew Hair Grooming Cream

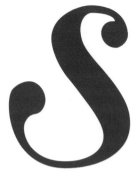

SO THERE YOU HAVE IT . . . TEN LOOKS TO LAST YOU A LIFETIME NO MATTER WHAT YOUR AGE, SIZE OR BODY SHAPE. So which look caught your fancy? Do you see yourself as a DISCO DIVA, BEATNIK BEAUTY or a wistful ROMANTIC HEROINE? Perhaps, like me, there's more than one style that appeals to you? I hope so. Being able to access a repertoire of looks will give you the confidence you need to shine in any situation.

No one is going to mess with a woman in a sharply Tailored outfit, or ignore a sassy Rock Chick. Fashion can be a very powerful tool to have at your disposal, especially if you're trying to stand out from the crowd and be noticed.

Spending time on your personal style is all about recapturing that sense of invincibility, the ability to turn heads and feel like the goddess you are inside. I hope this book becomes the personal stylist you always wished you had – a useful tool that liberates your sense of style and creativity, encouraging you to experiment with fresh new looks beyond your comfort zone.

May it be the beginning of a gorgeous, super-stylish new you!

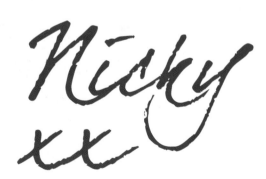

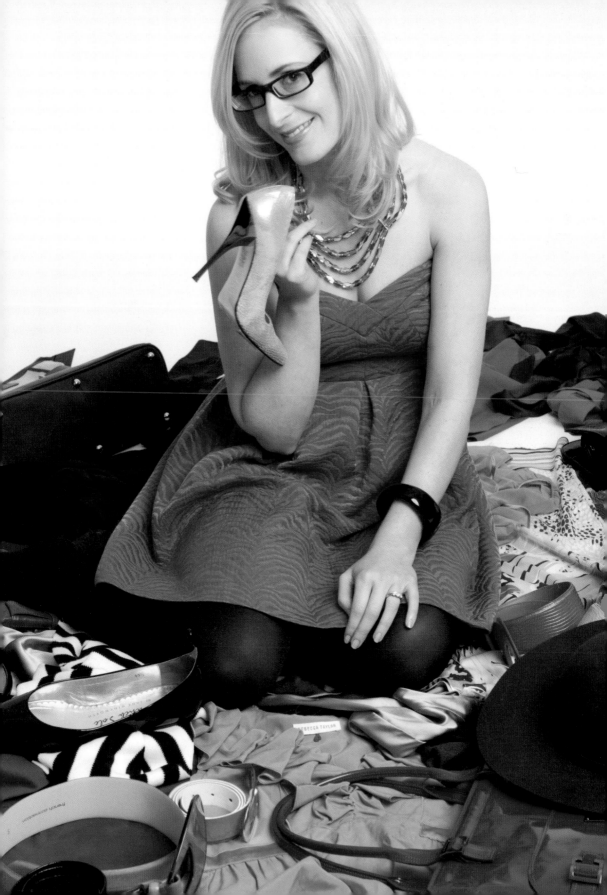

Index

INDEX

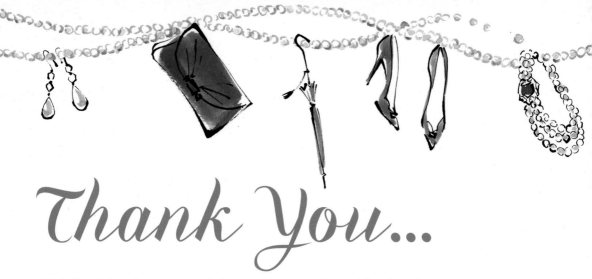

Thank You...

This book has been a real labour of love and wouldn't be the gorgeous book that it is without the help and support of some very special people.

✦ I'd firstly like to thank CLARE WATSON and KATIE ALLUM for helping me research the material for this book to the finest detail. Your input has been invaluable. Thank you for pulling out all the stops to ensure deadlines were met and I didn't go grey in the process.

✦ Thanks must also go to JULIAN ALEXANDER, my agent, who's stood by me through thick and thin. Thank you for all your support and guidance, which really helped to keep me focused and on track.

✦ To ZELDA TURNER, whose unfailing inspiration and passion for the book has transformed a black and white script into something that looks simply gorgeous.

✦ NIKKI DUPIN for her design talents which are second to none, a truly creative lady. I simply love the look and feel of the book – spot on!

✦ NEIL COOPER for being such a star photographer as always, ensuring we all look fresh as a daisy after a gruelling three-day shoot.

✦ NADIRA PERSAUD and MARIA KONIOS for the fabulous make-up on the shoot, as well a CLARE WATSON for sourcing clothes and styling the shoot.

✦ Last but not least, to CECILIA MOORE, TARA GLADDEN, ALICE WRIGHT, EMMA KNIGHT and all at HODDER who have played a part in getting the book to where it is today; it's been a truly consolidated team effort.